EMERGENCY
NURSING

EMERGENCY NURSING

An Essential Guide for Patient Care

Judy Selfridge-Thomas, MSN, RN, CEN, FNP

Selfridge, Sparger & Shea
Ventura, California
Nurse Practitioner
Department of Emergency Medicine
St. Mary Medical Center
Long Beach, California

W.B. SAUNDERS COMPANY

A Division of Harcourt Brace & Company

Philadelphia   London   Toronto   Montreal   Sydney   Tokyo

W.B. SAUNDERS COMPANY

A Division of Harcourt Brace & Company

The Curtis Center
Independence Square West
Philadelphia, Pennsylvania 19106

NOTICE

Emergency Nursing is an ever-changing field. Standard safety precautions must be followed, but as new research and clinical experience broaden our knowledge, changes in treatment and drug therapy become necessary or appropriate. The editors of this work have carefully checked the generic and trade drug names and verified drug dosages to ensure that the dosage information in this work is accurate and in accord with the standards accepted at the time of publication. Readers are advised, however, to check the product information currently provided by the manufacturer of each drug to be administered to be certain that changes have not been made in the recommended dose or in the contraindications for administration. This is of particular importance in regard to new or infrequently used drugs. It is the responsibility of the treating physician, relying on experience and knowledge of the patient, to determine dosages and the best treatment for the patient. The editors cannot be responsible for misuse or misapplication of the material in this work.

THE PUBLISHER

Library of Congress Cataloging–in–Publication Data

Selfridge-Thomas, Judy.
    Emergency nursing: an essential guide for patient care/Judy
Selfridge-Thomas.
      p.   cm.
    Includes bibliographical references.
    ISBN 0–7216–4703–0
    1. Emergency nursing. I. Title.
    [DNLM: 1. Emergency Nursing. WY 154 S465ea 1997]
  RT120.E4S43 1997
  610.73'61—dc20
  DNLM/DLC

96-23285

EMERGENCY NURSING

ISBN 0–7216–4703–0

Last digit is the print number: 9 8 7 6 5 4 3 2 1

"Hold a true friend with both your hands, for friendship is rarer than love."

Nigerian Proverb
Charles Peguy

To my ever-loving family and especially to one of my first nursing mentors and dearest friend —Anne. You helped teach me the spirit and love of life and were the true soul of emergency nursing. I will miss you forever.

Introduction

The spectrum of nursing is again in the process of evolution as the U.S. health care system strives to define and identify its constituency, purpose, and expected outcomes. With system mergers, proliferation of managed care organizations, increasing emphasis on a return to primary care, and cost containment measures, the roles of medicine and nursing are being redefined.

Nowhere is this more evident than in the emergency department setting. Within the past 5 years, many previously assigned emergency nursing positions have been reengineered into multiskilled positions, and there has been a recent expansion of the nurse practitioner role in the emergency department. This has produced an even greater blurring of traditional nursing roles, with nurses assuming increasing responsibility for managing patient care.

This text was designed to provide my experienced emergency nursing colleagues with the essential knowledge required for that expanding accountability. The most common patient problems encountered in the emergency setting are presented in a one-page format for ease of accessing information. Pertinent information related to a specific diagnosis is readily available and includes: *Etiology, Common Complaints, Nursing Diagnoses, Triage Rating, Related Factors, Assessments, Diagnostics, Interventions,* and *Disposition.* It is important to note that in the *Interventions* column, commonly used medications along with dose ranges are provided. These are intended as guidelines and conventionally represent the most cost-effective medications prescribed for a particular patient problem. Different medications with similar actions may be used depending on the physician, nurse practitioner, or hospital or insurance formulary.

As the author of *Emergency Nursing: An Essential Guide for Patient Care*, it is my desire that my emergency nursing colleagues will find this text a valuable resource in providing patient care to the ever increasing and diverse patient population whom we interact with daily.

Judy Selfridge-Thomas

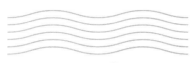

Contents

Life-Threatening Conditions

Anaphylactic Shock

Etiology
- Exposure to known or unknown allergen

Nursing Diagnoses
- Impaired gas exchange
- Altered tissue perfusion
- Decreased cardiac output

Common Complaints
- Coherent patient may complain of stridor, wheezing, abdominal cramps, diarrhea, swelling of lips or tongue, intense skin urticaria or pruritus.

Triage Rating
- Emergent

Related Factors
- Allergen may be a medication, food, or environmental substance. Reaction can occur up to 24 hours after exposure and may also display a biphasic pattern.

Assessment Findings
- Restlessness, decreasing level of consciousness, coma
- Respiratory stridor or possible respiratory arrest
- Angioedema
- Warm, flushed skin with possible urticaria rash
- Hypotension
- Tachycardia
- Incontinence

Diagnostics
- CBC: elevated WBC from cellular injury; elevated eosinophil and basophils
- ABG: pH <7.3 (metabolic acidosis), Pao_2 80–100 mm Hg, $Paco_2$ <30 mm Hg, (respiratory alkalosis)

Interventions
- Maintain patent airway: use airway adjuncts, possible intubation, or cricothyroidotomy procedures.
- Administer oxygen 6-15 L via face mask or bag-valve-mask device.
- Insert IV and infuse NS fluid.
- Obtain blood samples for CBC or other studies.
- Administer medications to impede further histamine release:
  - **Epinephrine** 0.5–1 mg IV or endotracheal tube 1:10,000; 0.3 mg (Peds: 0.01 mg/kg); SC 1:1000 may also be administered.
  - **Diphenhydramine** 50 mg (Peds: 2 mg/kg) IV/IM.
  - **Cimetidine** 300 mg IV infusion.
  - **Hydrocortisone** 100–250 mg IV *or* **methylprednisolone** 50–100 mg IV.
  - **Metaproterenol** 0.1–0.5 mL in 3–5 mL NS by nebulizer treatment.
- Consider insertion of nasogastric tube.
- Consider insertion of indwelling urinary catheter.
- Monitor level of consciousness, BP, pulse rate and rhythm, pulse oximetry, respiratory rate, stridor and respiratory wheezes, urinary output.

Disposition   Admission to critical care area.

Other   Recurrent episodes of anaphylaxis may occur 12–24 hours after the initial episode. Once the patient has recovered, education and prescribing of epinephrine kits for self-administration must be addressed.

Cardiogenic Shock

Etiology
- Recent myocardial infarction, trauma, cardiomyopathies

Nursing Diagnoses
- Decreased cardiac output
- Altered tissue perfusion
- Pain

Common Complaints
- Severe chest pain, sweating, shortness of breath

Triage Rating
- Emergent

Related Factors
- Any cause that reduces left ventricular ejection fraction (cardiac muscle damage, valvular dysfunction, tamponade) can lead to cardiogenic shock.

Assessment Findings
- Restlessness, decreasing level of consciousness
- Tachypnea
- Pulmonary rales
- Pale, diaphoretic skin
- Hypotension
- Cardiac dysrhythmias: bradycardia, tachycardia, PVCs
- Distended jugular veins or CVP >15 cm H_2O
- Possible S_3, S_4 heart sounds (muffled sounds if tamponade effect present)
- Reduced urine output

Diagnostics
- ECG: abnormal Q waves, elevated ST segment, dysrhythmias
- Cardiac enzymes: elevated CK and CK–MB isoenzyme

Interventions
- Administer oxygen 6–15 L via face mask or bag-valve-mask device.
- Consider transcutaneous external pacer machine.
- Insert IV and infuse NS fluid.
- Obtain blood samples for CBC, chemistries, cardiac enzymes, PT and PTT studies.
- Administer medications to maintain tissue perfusion and cardiac output and to reduce pain:
  - **Atropine sulfate** 0.5–1 mg to maximum of 0.04 mg/kg IV.
  - **Nitroglycerin** 0.04 mg SL or 5–20 µg/min IV infusion.
  - **Morphine sulfate** 2–4 mg increments IV.
  - **Antidysrhythmic** medication as required.*
  - **Sodium nitroprusside** 0.5–8 µg/kg/min IV infusion.
  - **Dopamine** or **dobutamine** 2–20 µg/kg/min IV infusion.
- Insert nasogastric tube and attach to suction.
- Insert indwelling urinary catheter.
- Assist with pericardiocentesis procedure if cause related to tamponade.
- Monitor level of consciousness, BP, pulse rate and rhythm, pulse oximetry, respiratory rate, pain relief, urine output.

*Administration of lidocaine may be necessary to reduce irritable ventricular foci: 1–1.5 mg/kg bolus repeated 5–10 minutes (0.5–0.75 mg/kg) to maximum dose of 3 mg/kg and a 2 g IV infusion of lidocaine at 2 mg/min may be required. Ventricular fibrillation is treated with defibrillation according to Advanced Cardiac Life Support (ACLS) guidelines.

Disposition
Admission to critical care area.

Hypovolemic Shock

Etiology
- Overt or covert volume loss

Nursing Diagnoses
- Fluid volume deficit
- Altered tissue perfusion
- Decreased cardiac output
- Impaired gas exchange

Common Complaints
- Coherent patients may complain of thirst, light-headedness, dizziness, vomiting, diarrhea, blood loss.

Triage Rating
- Emergent

Related Factors
- Condition associated with volume loss from injury; gastrointestinal, nasal, or vaginal bleeding; vomiting; diarrhea; major burns.

Asessment Findings
- Restlessness, decreasing level of consciousness, coma
- Pale, diaphoretic skin
- Hypotension: with narrowed (early compensation) or widened (uncompensated) pulse pressure
- Tachycardia
- Tachypnea
- Flattened jugular veins
- Possible visible injury, blood loss, emesis
- Reduced urine output

Diagnostics
- CBC: normal to low hemoglobin/hematocrit; WBC may be elevated from injury or stress
- ABG: pH <7.35 (metabolic acidosis), Pao_2 normal to <80 mm Hg, $Paco_2$ <30 mm Hg (respiratory alkalosis)
- Radiographic studies: chest, abdominal, extremity films; CT scan; ultrasound studies; arterial studies
- Possible peritoneal lavage procedure

Interventions
- Administer oxygen 6–15 L via face mask or bag-valve-mask device.
- Control external bleeding with direct pressure.
- Place patient in supine or modified V position.
- Insert IV and infuse fluid.*
- Obtain blood samples for CBC, chemistries, type and crossmatch, PT and PTT studies.
- Insert nasogastric tube and attach to suction.
- Insert indwelling urinary catheter.
- After volume restoration, administer vasopressor medication to maintain tissue perfusion: –**Dopamine** 2-10 µg/kg/min IV infusion not to exceed 50 µg/kg/min.
- Assist with invasive procedures: chest tube insertion, open thoracotomy.
- Infuse recovered blood from chest via autotransfusion.
- Monitor level of consciousness, BP, pulse rate and rhythm, pulse oximetry, respiratory rate, urinary output.

*Pediatric fluid infusion rate 20 mL/kg boluses (access may be via intraosseous route); resuscitation fluids can include NS, LR, hypertonic saline solution, hetastarch, albumin, Plasmanate, banked blood. Infusion rates dependent on fluid type and patient response.

Disposition   Admission to operating suite, critical care area, or if required transfer to regional trauma, burn, or pediatric center.

Neurogenic Shock

Etiology
- Spinal cord injury from trauma or recent spinal anesthesia

Nursing Diagnoses
- Altered tissue perfusion
- Decreased cardiac output

Common Complaints
- Decreased or diminished movement and sensation below level of injury

Triage Rating
- Emergent

Related Factors
- Condition requires high index of suspicion with associated neurologic, neck, and chest injuries.

Assessment Findings
- Restlessness, anxiety
- Warm, flushed skin
- Hypotension
- Bradycardia
- Tachypnea
- Decreased movement and sensation below level of injury
- Poor anal sphincter tone
- Possible urinary retention
- Development of poikilothermy

Diagnostics
- CBC: elevated WBC caused by injury
- ABG: pH <7.3 (metabolic acidosis), Pao_2 80–100 mm Hg, $Paco_2$ <30 mm Hg, (respiratory alkalosis)
- Radiographic studies:* cervical, thoracic, lumbar-sacral films; CT scan

Interventions
- Completely immobilize spinal column.
- Administer oxygen 6–15 L via face mask.
- Consider intubation because of development of respiratory fatigue.
- Insert IV and infuse NS fluid.
- Obtain blood samples for CBC, possible type and crossmatch, and other studies.
- Keep patient warm with blankets or warming lights.
- Consider administration of:
  –**Dopamine** dose higher than 10 µg/kg to obtain alpha effects.
  –**Methylprednisolone** if within 8 hours of injury, initial dose 30 mg/kg IV over 15 minutes, followed in 45 minutes with 5.4 mg/kg infusion over the next 23 hours.
- Insert nasogastric tube and attach to suction.
- Insert indwelling urinary catheter.
- Pad skeletal bony prominences.
- Assist with application of cervical traction as needed.
- Provide emotional support for patient and family.
- Monitor level of consciousness, BP, pulse rate and rhythm, pulse oximetry, respiratory rate, motor/sensory intactness, urinary output.

*Children are at risk for sustaining spinal cord injury without radiographic abnormality (SCIWORA).

Disposition   Admission to operating suite or critical care area, transfer to regional trauma or spinal cord injury center.

Septic Shock

Etiology
- Bacterial organism

Nursing Diagnoses
- Infection
- Altered tissue perfusion

Common Complaints
- Confusion, chills/fever

Triage Rating
- Emergent

Related Factors
- Associated with bacterial invasion, invasive procedure, or immune compromise and a common sequela of major traumatic injury. It is frequently a complication associated with the pediatric and elderly populations. The complication of disseminated intravascular coagulation (DIC) is high.

Assessment Findings
- Restlessness, decreasing level of consciousness
- Fever in early sepsis: subnormal temperature may be present in neonatal age group and in the elderly population
- Hypotension
- Tachycardia
- Skin may be warm, dry, and flushed; or may be cold and clammy; petechiae may be present

Diagnostics
- WBC: usually elevated with a left shift
- Coagulation studies: abnormal results include elevated fibrin degradation products, increased PT, decreased fibrinogen level, decreased platelets
- ABG: pH <7.3 (metabolic acidosis), PaO_2 normal to <80 mm Hg, $PaCO_2$ (variable)
- Radiographic studies: chest to determine if pneumonia is present
- Culture/sensitivity of urine, open wounds, sputum, blood
- Lumbar puncture: if meningitis is suspected, increased WBC, decreased glucose, increased protein, positive Gram's stain (gram-negative bacilli or rods)

Interventions
- Administer oxygen 6–15 L via face mask or bag-valve-mask device.
- Insert IV and infuse fluids.*
- Obtain blood samples for CBC coagulation profile, culture samples; culture samples from other sites as needed.
- Insert nasogastric tube and attach to suction.
- Insert indwelling urinary catheter.
- Administer antibiotic medication:†
  –**Ampicillin** 150–200 mg/kg/d IV/IM (Peds: 50–200 mg/kg/d) *or* **ampicillin sulbactam** 1.5–3 g IV infusion *plus* **gentamicin** 2 mg/kg IM/ IV infusion loading dose *or* **tobramycin** 2 mg/kg IM/IV infusion loading dose.
  –**Nafcillin** 1–2 g IM/IV infusion (Peds: 50–200 mg/kg qid) may also be added.
- Administer vasopressor medication to maintain tissue perfusion:
  –**Dopamine** 3-15 µg/kg/min IV infusion.
- Monitor level of consciousness, BP, pulse rate and rhythm, pulse oximetry, respiratory rate, urine output, core temperature.

*Pediatric fluid infusion rate 20 mL/kg bolus and may need to be as high as 60 mL/kg (access may be via intraosseous route); in adults volume replacement may be between 5 and 15 L.

†**Site of Infection** — **Suggested Antibiotic**

Site of Infection	Suggested Antibiotic
Gastrointestinal tract	**Ampicillin + gentamicin**
Respiratory tract	**Penicillin G** 20–24 million units IV infusion divided q4h or **clindamycin** 300–900 mg IV infusion (Peds: 8–40 mg/kg/d) –**Cefoxitin** 1–2 g IM/IV infusion or **cefazolin** 0.5–2 g IM/IV infusion may be substituted for **penicillin G + gentamicin**
Abdominal tract	**Clindamycin + gentamicin**
Skin/bone/joint	**Nafcillin, oxacillin** 1–2 g IM/IV infusion, or **methicillin** 1–2 g IM/IV infusion (Peds: 50 mg/kg/d) + **Gentamicin or clindamycin**
Immunocompromised host	**Ticarcillin** 3–4 g IV/IM (Peds: 200–300 mg/kg/d) + **gentamicin; cefotaxime** 1–2 g IV infusion (Peds: 50–180 mg/kg/d) may be added

Disposition Admission to critical care area or if required transfer to regional pediatric center.

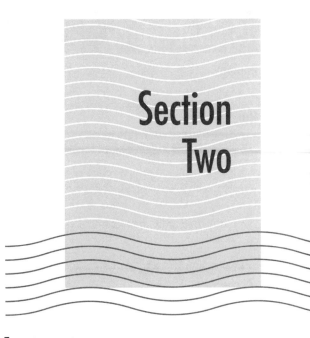

Section Two

Major System Injuries

Spinal Injury

Etiology
- Trauma

Nursing Diagnoses
- Risk for ineffective breathing
- Risk for decreased cardiac output
- Risk for altered urinary elimination
- Sensory/perception alteration
- Ineffective individual coping patterns

Common Complaints
- Loss of motor and sensory function below level of injury, numbness or tingling of extremities, inability to void or incontinence, pain

Triage Rating
- Urgent to emergent

Related Factors
- The majority of injuries are closed, with the mechanism of hyperflexion being the most common. Other mechanisms include hyperextension and axial loading. Penetrating injuries are rare. Injuries can involve only the vertebral bodies or complete or incomplete cord injury. The level of cord injury is determined by the lowest cord segment with sensory and motor function intactness.

Assessment Findings
- Injuries above C-3: respiratory arrest
- C-5, C-6 injury: diaphragm involvement; deltoid, biceps, and wrist extensors involved; sensation changes at thumb and first finger
- C-7: triceps involvement; sensation changes at third finger
- C-8, T-1: finger flexion and abduction involved; sensation changes at fourth and fifth fingers
- Incomplete lesions: deficit below level of injury:
  –Brown-Sequard—loss of motor function and contralateral loss of pain and temperature sensation
  –Central cord—both motor and sensory deficits with loss being greater in lower extremities
  –Anterior cord—loss of motor, pain, and temperature function
- Bony or muscle tenderness over area of injury
- Possible incontinence or urinary retention
- Possible saddle anesthesia

Diagnostics
- Radiographic studies: initial cross table lateral cervical spine (all seven cervical vertebrae must be visualized); possible flexion/extension views; thoracic-lumbar films; CT scan
- ABG: may be within normal limits or, depending on level of respiratory compromise, may indicate Pao_2 <80 mm Hg, $Paco_2$ >45 mm Hg (respiratory acidosis), pH <7.35 (acidosis)

Interventions
- Completely immobilize spinal column.
- Administer oxygen 6–15 L via face mask.
- Consider intubation if development of respiratory fatigue.
- Insert IV and infuse NS fluid.
- Consider obtaining ABG sample if respiratory involvement.
- Consider administration of pain medication:
  –**Meperidine** 25–100 mg IV/IM.
- Consider insertion of indwelling urinary catheter
- Assist with placement of cervical traction if unstable cervical fracture present.
- Monitor level of consciousness, BP, pulse rate and rhythm, pulse oximetry, respiratory rate, motor/sensory intactness, urinary output.

Disposition   Admission to operating suite or critical care area or transfer to regional trauma or spinal cord injury center unless injury is mild and does not involve bony fracture.

Cerebral Contusion

Etiology
- Trauma

Nursing Diagnoses
- Altered tissue perfusion: cerebral

Common Complaints
- Confusion, headache

Triage Rating
- Urgent to emergent

Related Factors
- Associated with high-velocity or acceleration/deceleration forces. Consists of petechial hemorrhage and fluid extravasation from injured vessels. Complications include cerebral ischemia, edema, increased ICP, and cerebral necrosis. Contrecoup injury opposite the point of impact is frequently present.

Assessment Findings
- Dependent on extent and location of injury
- Decreased level of consciousness, confusion
- Nausea/vomiting
- Speech dysfunction, personality and behavior changes, and motor deficits frequent

Diagnostics
- Radiographic studies: lateral cervical spine to determine coexisting injury
- CT scan: cerebral lesion with possible increased cerebral edema or structural shift

Interventions
- Maintain open and patent airway with adjuncts or possible intubation.*
- Continue cervical spine immobilization.
- Administer oxygen 6–15 L via face mask or bag-valve-mask device. Consider hyperventilation to produce initial cerebral vascular vasoconstriction.
- Insert IV and infuse fluids.†
- Obtain blood samples for CBC, alcohol level, and other studies.
- Consider administration of medications to decrease ICP:
  – **Mannitol** 0.25–1g/kg IV.
  – **Furosemide** 20–60 mg IV.
- Administer other prescribed medications:
  – **Phenytoin** loading dose to control seizure activity (controversial).
- Insert nasogastric tube and attach to suction.
- Consider insertion of indwelling urinary catheter.
- Consider insertion of ICP monitoring device.
- Monitor level of consciousness, BP, pulse rate and rhythm, respiratory rate, pulse oximeter, urinary output, ICP readings.
- Maintain head of bed at approximately 30 degrees if no concurrent spinal injury, neutral head alignment, and avoid activities that may increase ICP.

*Intubation procedure may require rapid sequenced induction with sedative and paralytic medications. Common medications include:
- **Midazolam** 1 mg slowly up to 5 mg IV
- **Morphine sulfate** 10 mg IV
- **Vecuronium** 0.1 mg/kg IV
- **Succinylcholine** 1–1.5 mg/kg IV (Peds: 2 mg/kg)
- **Pancuronium** 0.1 mg/kg IV

†Intravenous fluids must be infused at a rate to maintain vascular hemodynamics but not contribute to increased ICP.

Disposition
Admission to critical care area or if required transfer to regional center. Controversy exists whether operative intervention is required if a 5–7 mm shift is present on CT scan.

Subdural Hematoma

Etiology
- Trauma

Nursing Diagnoses
- Altered tissue perfusion: cerebral

Common Complaints
- Confusion, headache

Triage Rating
- Urgent to emergent

Related Factors
- A collection of venous blood beneath the dura. Classification determined according to onset of symptoms following injury: acute <48 hours, subacute within 48 hours–2 weeks, chronic >2 weeks. Elderly population and individuals with chronic alcoholism are prone to develop subacute or chronic hematomas. Child abuse must be considered in infants.

Assessment Findings
- Dependent on the extent of hematoma
- Decreased level of consciousness, confusion, irritability
- Nausea/vomiting
- Possible ipsilateral unequal pupil size and reaction
- Contralateral motor changes

Diagnostics
- Radiographic studies: lateral cervical spine to determine coexisting injury; CT scan indicating subdural location with possible structural shift

Interventions
- Maintain open and patent airway with adjuncts or possible intubation.*
- Continue cervical spine immobilization.
- Administer oxygen 6–15 L via face mask or bag-valve-mask device. Consider hyperventilation to produce initial cerebral vascular vasoconstriction.
- Insert IV and infuse fluids.†
- Obtain blood samples for CBC, possible alcohol level, or coagulation studies.
- Consider administration of medications to decrease ICP:
  –**Mannitol** 0.25–1 g/kg IV.
  –**Furosemide** 20–60 mg IV.
- Administer other prescribed medications:
  –**Phenytoin** loading dose to control seizure activity (controversial).
- Insert nasogastric tube and attach to suction.
- Consider insertion of indwelling urinary catheter.
- Monitor level of consciousness, BP, pulse rate and rhythm, respiratory rate, pulse oximeter, urinary output.
- Maintain head of bed at approximately 30 degrees if no concurrent spinal injury, neutral head alignment, and avoid activities that may increase ICP.

*Intubation procedure may require rapid sequenced induction with sedative and paralytic medications:
- **Midazolam** 1 mg slowly up to 5 mg IV
- **Morphine sulfate** up to 10 mg IV
- **Vecuronium** 0.1 mg/kg IV
- **Succinylcholine** 1–1.5 mg/kg IV (Peds: 2 mg/kg)
- **Pancuronium** 0.1 mg/kg IV

†IV fluids must be infused at a rate to maintain vascular hemodynamics but not contribute to increased ICP.

Disposition
Admission to operating suite for hematoma evacuation, admission to critical care area or if required transfer to regional center.

Epidural Hematoma

Etiology
- Trauma

Nursing Diagnoses
- Altered tissue perfusion: cerebral

Common Complaints
- Usually comatose, but may present with confusion or headache

Triage Rating
- Emergent

Related Factors
- Commonly the result of a tear or laceration of the middle or posterior meningeal artery. Frequently associated with a skull fracture. Usual sites are the temporal, frontal, and occipital cerebral regions.

Assessment Findings
- Decreased level of consciousness
- Initial presentation may involve an initial loss of consciousness (possibly caused by concussion), followed by a lucid period, with subsequent progression to unconsciousness (because of increased ICP)
- Possible ipsilateral unequal pupil size and reaction
- Contralateral motor changes or hemiparesis

Diagnostics
- Radiographic studies: lateral cervical spine to determine coexisting injury; CT scan indicating epidural location with possible structural shift

Interventions
- Maintain open and patent airway with adjuncts or possible intubation.*
- Continue cervical spine immobilization.
- Administer oxygen 6–15 L via face mask or bag-valve-mask device. Consider hyperventilation to produce initial cerebral vascular vasoconstriction.
- Insert IV and infuse fluids.†
- Obtain blood samples for CBC, possible alcohol level, or coagulation studies.
- Consider administration of medications to decrease ICP:
  –**Mannitol** 0.25–1 g/kg IV.
  –**Furosemide** 20–60 mg IV.
- Administer other prescribed medications:
  –**Phenytoin** loading dose to control seizure activity (controversial).
- Insert nasogastric tube and attach to suction.
- Consider insertion of indwelling urinary catheter.
- Monitor level of consciousness, BP, pulse rate and rhythm, respiratory rate, pulse oximeter, urinary output.
- Maintain head of bed at approximately 30 degrees if no concurrent spinal injury, neutral head alignment, and avoid activities that may increase ICP.

*Intubation procedure may require rapid sequence induction with sedative and paralytic medications:
- **Midazolam** 1 mg slowly up to 5 mg IV
- **Morphine sulfate** up to 10 mg IV
- **Vercuronium** 0.1 mg/kg IV
- **Succinylcholine** 1–1.5 mg/kg IV (Peds: 2 mg/kg)
- **Pancuronium** 0.1 mg/kg IV

†Intravenous fluids must be infused at a rate to maintain vascular hemodynamics but not contribute to increased ICP.

Disposition   Admission to operating suite for hematoma evacuation, or if required transfer to regional center.

Intracerebral Hemorrhage/Hematoma

Etiology
- Trauma, spontaneous bleeding

Nursing Diagnoses
- Altered tissue perfusion: cerebral

Common Complaints
- Confusion, headache

Triage Rating
- Emergent

Related Factors
- Involves bleeding into brain tissue and is frequently deep within the brain. Common sites involve frontal and temporal cerebral lobes. Hematomas may or may not be operable and are frequently associated with the development of cerebral edema.

Assessment Findings
- Dependent on the extent and location of the hemorrhage
- Decreased level of consciousness, confusion, irritability or possible coma
- Pupil reaction may range from normal to dilated and unreactive
- Progressive motor changes with possible hemiparesis

Diagnostics
- Radiographic studies: lateral cervical spine to determine coexisting injury; CT scan indicating hemorrhage or hematoma location and possible structural shifting

Interventions
- Maintain open and patent airway with adjuncts or possible intubation.*
- Continue cervical spine immobilization.
- Administer oxygen 6–15 L via face mask or bag-valve-mask device. Consider hyperventilation to produce initial cerebral vascular vasoconstriction.
- Insert IV and infuse fluids.†
- Obtain blood samples for CBC, possible alcohol level, or coagulation studies.
- Consider administration of medications to decrease ICP:
  –**Mannitol** 0.25–1g/kg IV.
  –**Furosemide** 20–60 mg IV.
- Administer other prescribed medications:
  –**Phenytoin** loading dose to control seizure activity (controversial).
- Insert nasogastric tube and attach to suction.
- Consider insertion of indwelling urinary catheter.
- Monitor level of consciousness, BP, pulse rate and rhythm, respiratory rate, pulse oximeter, urinary output.
- Maintain head of bed at approximately 30 degrees if no concurrent spinal injury, neutral head alignment, and avoid activities that may increase ICP.

*Intubation procedure may require rapid sequence induction with sedative and paralytic medications:
- **Midazolam** 1 mg slowly up to 5 mg IV
- **Morphine sulfate** up to 10 mg IV
- **Vercuronium** 0.1 mg/kg IV
- **Succinylcholine** 1–1.5 mg/kg IV (Peds: 2 mg/kg)
- **Pancuronium** 0.1 mg/kg IV

†Intravenous fluids must be infused at a rate to maintain vascular hemodynamics but not contribute to increased ICP.

Disposition   Admission to critical care area, or possibly the operating suite for hematoma evacuation, or if required transfer to regional center.

Subarachnoid Hemorrhage/Aneurysm Rupture

Etiology
- Thinning of a cerebral arterial wall, advanced atherosclerosis or infected emboli

Nursing Diagnoses
- Altered tissue perfusion: cerebral

Common Complaints
- Usually comatose, but may have confusion, severe headache

Triage Rating
- Emergent

Related Factors
- Rupture may be precipitated by heavy lifting or exercise or a hypertensive event. Blood in the subarachnoid space is chemically irritating and produces meningeal signs.

Assessment Findings
- Dependent on the extent of bleeding into the subarachnoid space. Graded from 1–5 (1 indicates minimal bleeding; 5 indicates severe bleeding)
- Sudden onset of severe or different type of usual headache
- Nausea/vomiting
- Photophobia
- Decreasing level of consciousness, confusion, irritability, or possible coma
- Nuchal rigidity
- Focal deficits: mild motor, speech, visual changes; or hemiparesis; or decerebrate posturing

Diagnostics
- Radiographic studies: CT scan indicating presence of blood in subarachnoid space with possible structural shifts; possible angiography
- Possible lumbar puncture with finding of blood in CSF and increased opening pressures **–CAUTION: Not to be performed in patients with suspected bleeding grades 3–5 until after CT results**
- ECG changes may indicate T wave changes of elevation, depression, or inversion; U waves may be present

Interventions
- Maintain open and patent airway with adjuncts or possible intubation.
- Administer oxygen 6–15 L via face mask or bag-valve-mask device. Hyperventilation after intubation may be required to produce initial cerebral vascular vasoconstriction.
- Insert IV and infuse minimal NS fluid.
- Obtain blood samples for CBC, coagulation profile.
- Administer medications:
  –Diazepam 5–10 mg IV.
  –Nimodipine 60 mg PO.
- Insert nasogastric tube and attach to suction.
- Consider insertion of indwelling urinary catheter.
- Monitor level of consciousness, BP, pulse rate and rhythm, respiratory rate, pulse oximeter, urinary output.
- Maintain head of bed at approximately 30 degrees, neutral head alignment, and avoid activities that may increase ICP.

Disposition   Admission to critical care area or possibly operating suite for surgical clipping of aneurysm.

Mandibular Fracture

Etiology
- Trauma

Nursing Diagnoses
- Pain
- Sensory/perceptual alteration
- Risk for ineffective airway clearance

Common Complaints
- Jaw pain in association with mal-occlusion, drooling, and possible numbness of the lower lip

Triage Rating
- Urgent to emergent

Related Factors
- Direct blunt force to the mandibular bone is the most common mechanism of injury. Additional injuries may include mandibular contusion, hematoma, or intraoral laceration.

Assessment Findings
- Swelling, asymmetry of mandible
- Trismus
- Oral bleeding
- Possible drooling
- Possible ruptured tympanic membrane or hemotympanum on side of injury
- Palpable pain over injury site
- Decreased or altered sensation on affected side

Diagnostics
- Radiographic studies: mandibular, Panorex films; CT scan

Interventions
- Position patient in high-Fowler's position if no concurrent spinal injury.
- Suction oral cavity to prevent secretions or blood from pooling and causing airway obstruction.
- Consider insertion of IV or saline lock.
- Administer medications to decrease pain:
  –**Meperidine** 25–100 mg IV/IM *or* **morphine sulfate** 2–4 mg IV then titrated to achieve pain relief *or* **acetaminophen with codeine** *or* **hydrocodone** PO.
- Administer antibiotic medications for open fractures:
  –**Procaine penicillin** 2–4 million units IM followed by PO dose
  –**Penicillin V** 500 mg PO qid × 7 5–7 days *or* **aqueous penicillin G** 10–12 million units IV divided q4–6h.
- Administer **dT** 0.5 mL IM if necessary.
- Assist with application of arch bars for fracture stabilization.
- Monitor airway patency, BP, pulse rate and rhythm, pulse oximetry, respiratory rate, pain relief.

Disposition
Admission to operating suite or hospitalization should be considered for patients with severely displaced or open fractures. Other patients may be released to home with referral to an oral surgeon, plastic surgeon, or otolaryngologist. Provide instructions to increase fluid intake using a straw or to eat only soft foods for 24–48 hours.

Maxillary Fracture

Etiology
- Trauma

Nursing Diagnoses
- Pain
- Sensory/perceptual alteration
- Risk for ineffective airway clearance

Common Complaints
- Midfacial pain, possible visual changes (diplopia), nasal bleeding

Triage Rating
- Urgent to emergent

Related Factors
- Direct blunt force to the maxillary bone is the most common mechanism of injury. Fractures are classified according to fracture lines: Le Fort I (horizontal fracture); Le Fort II (pyramidal fracture); Le Fort III (complete cranial/facial separation). Other system injuries may also be present.

Assessment Findings
- Facial swelling over fracture site
- Facial asymmetry
- Oral/nasal bleeding or possible CSF drainage from nose or ears
- Palpable pain over injury site
- Facial mobility:
  - I—lower maxilla
  - II—nasal/dental arch
  - III—craniofacial separation

Diagnostics
- Radiographic studies: facial series, CT scan

Interventions
- Position patient in high-Fowler's position if no concurrent spinal injury.
- Suction oral cavity to prevent secretions or blood from pooling and causing airway obstruction.
- Assist with possible intubation or cricothyroidotomy to maintain airway patency.
- Insert IV and infuse NS fluid for Le Fort II and III injuries.
- Obtain blood samples for CBC, chemistries, type and crossmatch, PT and PTT studies.
- Insert orogastric tube and attach to suction.
- Insert indwelling urinary catheter if volume resuscitation is required.
- Administer medications to decrease pain:
  - **Meperidine** 25–100 mg IM/IV *or* **morphine sulfate** 2–4 mg IV and titrated to achieve pain relief *or* **acetaminophen with codeine** *or* **hydrocodone** PO.
- Administer antibiotic medications for open fracture:
  - **Procaine penicillin** 2–4 million units IM followed by oral dose of **penicillin V potassium** 500 mg PO qid × 5–7 days *or* **aqueous penicillin G** 10–12 million units IV divided q4–6h.
- Administer **dT** 0.5 mL IM if necessary.
- Monitor airway patency, BP, pulse rate and rhythm, pulse oximetry, respiratory rate, pain relief.

Disposition   Admission to operating suite or hospitalization for patients with Le Fort II or III fractures. Patients with Le Fort I fractures may be released to home with referral to an oral surgeon, plastic surgeon, or otolaryngologist. Provide instructions to increase fluid intake using a straw or to eat only soft foods for 24–48 hours.

Tracheobronchial Tree Injury

Etiology
- Trauma

Nursing Diagnoses
- Ineffective airway clearance
- Ineffective breathing pattern
- Impaired gas exchange

Common Complaints
- Pain, shortness of breath

Triage Rating
- Emergent

Related Factors
- Most common areas of injury are the distal trachea or proximal main stem bronchi.

Assessment Findings
- Stridor
- Cyanosis
- Intercostal muscle use
- Intercostal retractions
- Subcutaneous emphysema in the area of injury
- Oxygen saturation <94%
- Decreased breath sounds if pneumothorax is present
- Hemoptysis

Diagnostics
- Radiographic studies: chest films may identify concurrent pneumothorax
- Bronchoscopy: will identify area of injury

Interventions
- Suction airway to maintain patency.
- Administer oxygen 6–15 L via face mask.
- Assist with intubation procedure or cricothyrotomy.
- Assist with chest tube insertion if concurrent pneumothorax is present.
- Insert IV and infuse NS fluids.
- Insert nasogastric tube and attach to suction.
- Insert indwelling urinary catheter.
- Monitor airway patency, level of consciousness, BP, pulse rate and rhythm, pulse oximetry, respiratory rate, urinary output.

Disposition   Admission to operating suite for surgical repair.

Cardiac Contusion

Etiology
- Trauma

Nursing Diagnoses
- Decreased cardiac output
- Altered tissue perfusion
- Pain

Common Complaints
- Chest pain

Triage Rating
- Urgent to emergent

Related Factors
- Occurs from blunt force injury to the thorax. Contusion of the right ventricle occurs more frequently than to the left ventricle. May precipitate a myocardial infarction in persons with preexisting coronary artery disease.

Assessment Findings
- Possible ecchymosis on chest wall
- Possible tachycardia
- Possible hypotension
- Possible distended jugular veins or CVP >15 cm H_2O
- Possible S_3 and S_4 heart sounds
- Possible pale, diaphoretic skin

Diagnostics
- ECG: may be normal or may indicate nonspecific to elevated ST segments, dysrhythmias
- Cardiac enzymes: elevated CK and CK–MB isoenzyme
- Echocardiography: wall motion abnormalities may be identified

Interventions
- Administer oxygen 6–15 L via face mask.
- Insert IV and infuse fluids.*
- Obtain blood samples for CBC, cardiac enzymes, PT and PTT studies.
- Administer medications to treat dysrhythmias[†] and reduce pain:
  – **Morphine sulfate** 2–4 mg IV initially, then titrated to continue pain relief.
- Consider insertion of nasogastric tube and attach to suction.
- Consider insertion of indwelling urinary catheter.
- Monitor level of consciousness, BP, pulse rate and rhythm, pulse oximetry, pain relief.

*Infuse fluids of NS but do not overload damaged myocardium.
[†]Administration of **lidocaine** may be necessary to reduce irritable ventricular foci: 1–1.5 mg/kg bolus repeated q 5–10min (0.5–0.75 mg/kg) to maximum dose of 3 mg/kg and a 2 g IV infusion of **lidocaine** at 2 mg/min may be required.

Disposition Admission to critical care area for observation.

Open Pneumothorax

Etiology
- Trauma

Nursing Diagnoses
- Ineffective breathing pattern
- Impaired gas exchange
- Risk for fluid volume deficit

Common Complaints
- Difficulty breathing, chest pain from injury forces

Triage Rating
- Emergent

Related Factors
- Penetrating injury to the thorax may result in both an open pneumothorax and a hemothorax.

Assessment Findings
- Cyanosis
- Obvious open chest wound with possible bubbling of fluids
- Trachypnea with increased respiratory effort
- Oxygen saturation <94%
- Decreased breath sounds and hyperresonant percussion sounds on affected side

Diagnostics
- Radiographic studies: chest films indicating size and location of pneumothorax

Interventions
- Administer oxygen 6–15 L via face mask or bag-valve-mask device.
- Cover open wound using occlusive dressing taped on three sides.*
- Assist with chest tube insertion procedure and consider autotransfusion if concurrent hemothorax is present.
- Insert IV and infuse fluids.†
- Obtain blood samples for CBC, chemistries, type and crossmatch, PT and PTT studies.
- Consider insertion of nasogastric tube and attach to suction.
- Insert indwelling urinary catheter.
- Administer **dT** 0.5 mL IM if necessary.
- Monitor level of consciousness, BP, pulse rate and rhythm, pulse oximetry, respiratory rate, urinary output.

*If tension pneumothorax develops, remove occlusive dressing.
†Resuscitation fluids may include NS, LR, hetastarch, albumin, Plasmanate, or autotransfused or banked blood. Infusion rates depend on patient response.

Disposition   Admission to operating suite or critical care area or if required transfer to regional trauma center.

Tension Pneumothorax

Etiology
- Trauma

Nursing Diagnoses
- Ineffective breathing pattern
- Impaired gas exchange
- Risk for ineffective airway clearance

Common Complaints
- Sudden worsening of ability to breathe, associated pain resulting from injury forces

Triage Rating
- Emergent

Related Factors
- Air collection in the thoracic cavity can lead to compression of mediastinal structures, resulting in rapid progression to death.

Assessment Findings
- Restlessness
- Extreme tachypnea
- Cyanosis
- Distended jugular veins
- Hypotension
- Tachycardia
- Oxygen saturation <94%
- Decreased breath sounds and hyperresonant percussion sounds on affected side
- Tracheal deviation toward unaffected side
- Displaced and distant heart sounds

Diagnostics
- Radiographic studies: chest films demonstrate size and location of pneumothorax

Interventions
- Administer oxygen 6–15 L via face mask.
- Assist with immediate chest decompression using a large gauge needle or chest tube.
- Insert IV and infuse NS fluids.
- Consider insertion of nasogastric tube and attach to suction.
- Consider insertion of indwelling urinary catheter.
- Monitor level of consciousness, BP, pulse rate and rhythm, pulse oximetry, respiratory rate, urinary output.

Disposition   Admission to critical care area.

Hemothorax

Etiology
- Trauma

Nursing Diagnoses
- Fluid volume deficit
- Altered tissue perfusion
- Decreased cardiac output
- Ineffective breathing pattern
- Impaired gas exchange

Common Complaints
- Conscious patients may complain of increasing respiratory difficulty and pain

Triage Rating
- Emergent

Related Factors
- Penetrating or blunt forces to the thorax may result in a hemothorax. Depending on the volume of blood sequestered in the thoracic cavity, a hemothorax is classified as mild (<500 mL) to major (>2500 mL). Autotransfusion procedure should be considered.

Assessment Findings
- Restlessness, decreasing level of consciousness
- Pale, diaphoretic skin
- Hypotension
- Tachycardia
- Tachypnea
- Oxygen saturation <94%
- Diminished/absent breath sounds and dull percussion sounds on affected side
- Flattened jugular veins

Diagnostics
- CBC: normal to low hemoglobin/hematocrit level; possible elevated WBC from injury
- Radiographic studies: chest films demonstrating size and location of hemothorax
- Obvious blood return from inserted chest tube

Interventions
- Administer oxygen 6–15 L via face mask.
- Assist with chest tube insertion and possible autotransfusion.
- Insert IV and infuse fluids.*
- Obtain blood samples for CBC, chemistries, type and crossmatch, PT and PTT studies.
- Assist with open thoracotomy procedure as indicated.
- Insert nasogastric tube and attach to suction.
- Insert indwelling urinary catheter.
- Administer **dT** 0.5 mL IM if necessary.
- Monitor level of consciousness, BP, pulse rate and rhythm, pulse oximetry, respiratory rate, chest tube fluid output, urinary output.

*Resuscitation fluids may include NS, LR, autotransfused or banked blood, hetastarch, albumin, or Plasmanate. Infusion rates depend on patient response.

Disposition   Admission to operating suite or critical care area or if required transfer to regional trauma center.

Flail Chest

Etiology
- Trauma

Nursing Diagnoses
- Ineffective breathing pattern
- Impaired gas exchange
- Pain

Common Complaints
- Pain with increasing difficulty breathing

Triage Rating
- Emergent

Related Factors
- Blunt injury forces are responsible for a flail chest. It is common for other system injuries to be present also. Pulmonary contusion are commonly associated with a flail chest. Adult respiratory distress syndrome (ARDS) frequently develops within hours to days after the initial injury.

Assessment Findings
- Increased restlessness
- Extreme difficulty breathing
- Cyanosis
- Tachypnea along with shallow respirations
- Oxygen saturation <94%
- Possible asymmetry of chest wall motion
- Crepitus over injured area

Diagnostics
- Radiographic studies: chest films indicating fracture of two or more ribs in two or more places on the same side or a free-floating sternum
- ABG: pH <7.3 (acidosis), $Paco_2$ >45 mm Hg (respiratory acidosis), HCO_3 normal, Pao_2 <80 mm Hg

Interventions
- Administer oxygen 6–15 L via face mask or bag-valve-mask device.
- Assist with intubation and mechanical ventilation.
- Insert IV and infuse fluids.*
- Obtain blood samples for CBC, chemistries, type and crossmatch, PT and PTT studies.
- Insert nasogastric tube and attach to suction.
- Insert indwelling urinary catheter.
- Consider pain control via administration of **bupivacaine (Marcaine)** as an intercostal block.
- Monitor level of consciousness, BP, pulse rate and rhythm, pulse oximetry, respiratory rate, urinary output.

*Resuscitation fluids can include NS, LR, or colloid fluids; however, care must be taken to maintain hemodymanic stability without overhydration. This is to minimize compounding an ARDS complication.

Disposition   Admission to critical care area or if required transfer to regional trauma center.

Liver Injury

Etiology
- Trauma

Nursing Diagnoses
- Fluid volume deficit
- Pain

Common Complaints
- Lower right-sided chest pain if rib involvement, right-sided abdominal pain, possible right shoulder pain

Triage Rating
- Urgent to emergent

Related Factors
- Injury forces may be blunt or penetrating and commonly involve high velocity acceleration/deceleration steering-wheel injury. The liver capsule may rupture, causing rapid blood loss and peritoneal contamination; whereas a subcapsular injury may not produce signs/symptoms until 72 hours after injury.

Assessment Findings
- Restlessness because of volume loss
- Hypotension
- Tachycardia
- Pale, diaphoretic skin
- Possible open wound on abdomen or ecchymoses of right upper abdominal quadrant
- Increasing right upper abdominal quadrant pain
- Decreasing bowel sounds
- Abdominal guarding, rebound tenderness, rigidity

Diagnostics
- Peritoneal lavage: presence of blood in returned fluid
- Radiographic studies: CT scan or ultrasound of abdomen indicating extent of injury
- CBC: normal to low hemoglobin/hematocrit level; possible elevated WBC from injury

Interventions
- Administer oxygen 6–15 L via face mask.
- Stabilize any impaled objects in chest/abdomen.
- Place patient in supine or modified V position.
- Insert IV and infuse fluids.*
- Obtain blood samples for CBC, chemistries, type and crossmatch, PT and PTT studies.
- Insert nasogastric tube and attach to suction.
- Insert indwelling urinary catheter.
- Monitor level of consciousness, BP, pulse rate and rhythm, pulse oximetry, respiratory rate, intensity of abdominal pain, urinary output.

*Pediatric fluid infusion rate is 20 mL/kg boluses; resuscitation fluids can include NS, LR, or colloid fluids. Infusion rates are dependent on fluid type and patient response.

Disposition   Admission to operating suite or critical care area or if required transfer to regional trauma or pediatric center.

Spleen Injury

Etiology
- Trauma

Nursing Diagnoses
- Fluid volume deficit
- Pain

Common Complaints
- Lower left-sided chest pain if rib involvement, left-sided abdominal pain, possible left shoulder pain

Triage Rating
- Urgent to emergent

Related Factors
- Injury forces may be blunt or penetrating. Conditions such as pregnancy, recent mononucleosis, leukemia, and sickle cell disease result in splenic enlargement, thus increasing organ injury risk. Mortality is related to hemorrhage from initial or delayed rupture, sepsis, or the development of postsplenectomy infection (OPSI). OPSI is often caused by pneumococci, therefore it is important that postsplenectomy patients receive polyvalent pneumococci vaccine.

Assessment Findings
- Restlessness because of volume loss
- Hypotension
- Tachycardia
- Pale, diaphoretic skin
- Possible open wound on abdomen or ecchymoses of left upper abdominal quadrant
- Increasing left upper abdominal quadrant pain
- Decreasing bowel sounds
- Abdominal guarding, rebound tenderness, rigidity
- Possible enlarging area of left flank dullness with percussion

Diagnostics
- Peritoneal lavage: presence of blood in returned fluid
- Radiographic studies: CT scan or ultrasound of abdomen indicating extent of injury
- CBC: normal to low hemoglobin/hematocrit level; possible elevated WBC from injury

Interventions
- Administer oxygen 6–15 L via face mask.
- Stabilize any impaled objects in chest/abdomen.
- Place patient in supine or modified V position.
- Insert IV and infuse fluids.*
- Obtain blood samples for CBC, chemistries, type and crossmatch, PT and PTT studies.
- Insert nasogastric tube and attach to suction.
- Insert indwelling urinary catheter.
- Monitor level of consciousness, BP, pulse rate and rhythm, pulse oximetry, respiratory rate, intensity of abdominal pain, urinary output.

*Pediatric fluid infusion rate is 20 mL/kg boluses; resuscitation fluids can include NS, LR, or colloid fluids. Infusion rates are dependent on fluid type and patient response.

Disposition   Admission to operating suite or critical care area or if required transfer to regional trauma or pediatric center.

Stomach Injury

Etiology
- Trauma

Nursing Diagnoses
- Pain
- Risk for infection

Common Complaints
- Epigastric abdominal pain, fever

Triage Rating
- Emergent

Related Factors
- Although the stomach is well protected from injury, either blunt or penetrating forces may result in a tear or rupture of the organ.

Assessment Findings
- Restlessness because of volume loss or pain
- Tachycardia
- Pale, diaphoretic skin
- Possible open wound on upper abdomen
- Increasing epigastric abdominal pain
- Decreasing bowel sounds
- Abdominal guarding, rebound tenderness, rigidity

Diagnostics
- Peritoneal lavage: presence of gastric fluid or undigested food
- Radiographic studies: CT scan or ultrasound of abdomen indicating extent of injury
- CBC: normal to low hemoglobin/hematocrit level; possible elevated WBC from injury

Interventions
- Administer oxygen 6–15 L via face mask.
- Stabilize any impaled objects in chest/abdomen.
- Place patient in supine or modified V position.
- Insert IV and infuse fluids.*
- Obtain blood samples for CBC, chemistries, type and crossmatch, PT and PTT studies.
- Insert nasogastric tube and attach to suction.
- Insert indwelling urinary catheter.
- Monitor level of consciousness, BP, pulse rate and rhythm, pulse oximetry, respiratory rate, intensity of abdominal pain, urinary output.

*Pediatric fluid infusion rate is 20 mL/kg boluses; resuscitation fluids can include NS, LR, or colloid fluids. Infusion rates are dependent on fluid type and patient response.

Disposition Admission to operating suite or critical care area or if required transfer to regional trauma or pediatric center.

Pancreatic Injury

Etiology
- Trauma

Nursing Diagnoses
- Fluid volume deficit
- Pain

Common Complaints
- Few indicators that reveal pancreatic injury is present other than epigastric pain

Triage Rating
- Urgent to emergent

Related Factors
- The majority of injury forces that cause pancreatic injury are penetrating. This injury carries a high mortality rate because of the high probability of additional associated intraabdominal injuries.

Assessment Findings
- Restlessness because of volume loss or pain
- Hypotension
- Tachycardia
- Pale, diaphoretic skin
- Possible open wound on abdomen or ecchymoses around the umbilicus
- Increasing epigastric pain
- Decreasing bowel sounds
- Abdominal guarding, rebound tenderness, rigidity

Diagnostics
- Peritoneal lavage: presence of blood, amylase, or lipase in returned fluid
- Radiographic studies: CT scan or ultrasound of abdomen indicating extent of injury
- CBC: normal to low hemoglobin/hematocrit level; possible elevated WBC from injury
- Serum amylase or lipase: elevated

Interventions
- Administer oxygen 6–15 L via face mask.
- Stabilize any impaled objects in chest/abdomen.
- Place patient in supine or modified V position.
- Insert IV and infuse fluids.*
- Obtain blood samples for CBC, chemistries, amylase, lipase, type and crossmatch, PT and PTT studies.
- Insert nasogastric tube and attach to suction.
- Insert indwelling urinary catheter.
- Monitor level of consciousness, BP, pulse rate and rhythm, pulse oximetry, respiratory rate, intensity of abdominal pain, urinary pain.

*Pediatric fluid infusion rate is 20 mL/kg boluses; resuscitation fluids can include NS, LR, or colloid fluids. Infusion rates are dependent on fluid type and patient response.

Disposition   Admission to operating suite or critical care area or if required transfer to regional trauma or pediatric center.

Bowel/Colon Injuries

Etiology
- Trauma

Nursing Diagnoses
- Fluid volume deficit
- Pain
- Risk for infection

Common Complaints
- Abdominal pain, emesis, fever

Triage Rating
- Urgent to emergent

Related Factors
- Injury may occur from either blunt or penetrating forces. Small bowel injuries are more likely to occur in patients who wear lap seat belts incorrectly (above the iliac crest). Penetrating forces result more frequently in colon injuries.

Assessment Findings
- Restlessness because of volume loss or pain
- Hypotension
- Tachycardia
- Pale, diaphoretic skin
- Possible open wounds or ecchymoses of abdomen or rectal area
- Increasing abdominal pain
- Distended abdomen
- Decreasing bowel sounds
- Abdominal guarding, rebound tenderness, rigidity
- Rectal bleeding

Diagnostics
- Radiographic studies: CT or ultrasound of abdomen indicating extent of injury
- CBC: normal to low hemoglobin/hematocrit level; possible elevated WBC from injury or infection
- Stool guaiac: positive for blood

Interventions
- Administer oxygen 6–15 L via face mask.
- Stabilize any impaled object in chest/abdomen.
- Place patient in supine or modified V position.
- Insert IV and infuse NS fluids.
- Obtain blood samples for CBC, chemistries, type and crossmatch, PT and PTT studies.
- Insert nasogastric tube and attach to suction.
- Insert indwelling urinary catheter.
- Monitor level of consciousness, BP, pulse rate and rhythm, pulse oximetry, respiratory rate, intensity of abdominal pain, urinary output.

Disposition   Admission to operating suite or critical care area or if required transfer to regional trauma center.

Renal Injuries

Etiology
- Trauma

Nursing Diagnoses
- Fluid volume deficit
- Pain
- Altered urinary elimination

Common Complaints
- Pain, emesis

Triage Rating
- Urgent to emergent

Related Factors
- Direct blows to the flank area or rapid deceleration mechanisms are frequently the cause of renal injury. Injury can range from mild contusions to severe cortical disruption.

Assessment Findings
- Restlessness because of volume loss or pain
- Hypotension if significant volume loss
- Tachycardia if significant volume loss
- Possible open wounds or ecchymoses on flank or lower posterior thorax area
- Decreased bowel sounds

Diagnostics
- Urinalysis: hematuria may be present or absent
- Radiographic studies: IVP, CT scan, or ultrasound of kidneys indicating site and extent of injury
- CBC: normal to low hemoglobin/hematocrit level; possible elevated WBC from injury

Interventions
- Administer oxygen 6–15 L via face mask.
- Stabilize any impaled object in chest/flank/abdomen.
- Insert IV and infuse NS fluids.
- Obtain blood samples for CBC, chemistries, type and crossmatch, PT and PTT studies.
- Insert nasogastric tube and attach to suction.
- Insert indwelling urinary catheter if no blood at the urinary meatus.
- Monitor level of consciousness, BP, pulse rate and rhythm, pulse oximetry, respiratory rate, intensity of abdominal pain, urinary output.

Disposition Admission to operating suite or critical care area or if required transfer to regional trauma center.

Bladder Injury

Etiology
- Trauma

Nursing Diagnoses
- Pain
- Altered urinary elimination

Common Complaints
- Abdominal or shoulder pain (if urine is present in the peritoneal cavity), inability to void, urinary frequency, nausea/vomiting

Triage Rating
- Urgent to emergent

Related Factors
- Occurs most frequently when the bladder is distended. Direct blows to the abdomen or a high-riding seat belt if involved in a motor vehicle crash are common injury mechanisms. Pelvic fractures can result in bladder injury, with the bladder dome being the most common site of rupture.

Assessment Findings
- Restlessness because of pain or volume loss
- Hypotension if significant volume loss
- Tachycardia because of pain or volume loss
- Suprapubic mass or tenderness
- Abdominal distension

Diagnostics
- Urinalysis: hematuria, either gross or microscopic
- Radiographic studies: cystogram, IVP, ultrasound, CT scan of bladder indicating injury or urine extravasation
- CBC: normal to low hemoglobin/hematocrit level; possible elevated WBC from injury

Interventions
- Administer oxygen 6–15 L via face mask.
- Insert IV and infuse NS fluids.
- Obtain blood samples for CBC, chemistries, type and crossmatch.
- Insert nasogastric tube and attach to suction.
- Insert indwelling urinary catheter if no blood at the urinary meatus.
- Monitor level of consciousness, BP, pulse rate and rhythm, pulse oximetry, respiratory rate, urinary output.

Disposition   Admission to operating suite or critical care area or if required transfer to regional trauma center.

Urethral Injury

Etiology
- Trauma

Nursing Diagnoses
- Pain
- Altered urinary elimination

Common Complaints
- Perineal pain, inability to void

Triage Rating
- Urgent to emergent

Related Factors
- Occurs more frequently in males than females. An anterior urethral injury is often associated with straddle-type injury, whereas posterior urethral injury is associated with pelvic fracture. In females, this injury is more likely to occur in children than adults and can be caused by direct injury or foreign object insertion.

Assessment Findings
- Blood at the urinary meatus
- Swelling of the scrotum, penis, or lower abdomen
- Butterfly pattern of ecchymosis below the scrotum with straddle-type injury
- Displaced prostate gland

Diagnostics
- Urinalysis: hematuria may be present
- Radiographic studies: retrograde urethrogram (before the insertion of an indwelling urinary catheter), IVP, CT scan, abdominal or pelvic radiographs, or cystogram indicating site and extent of injury
- CBC: normal to low hemoglobin/hematocrit level; possible elevated WBC from injury

Interventions
- Administer oxygen 6–15 L via face mask.
- Insert IV and infuse NS fluids.
- Obtain blood samples for CBC, chemistries, type and crossmatch.
- Monitor urinary output.*
- Monitor level of consciousness, BP, pulse rate and rhythm, pulse oximetry, respiratory rate.

*Placement of an indwelling urinary catheter to monitor urinary output is contraindicated if blood is present at the urinary meatus. A suprapubic catheter may be used to divert urine from the injured area.

Disposition   Admission to operating suite or critical care area or if required transfer to regional trauma center.

Pelvic Fracture

Etiology
- Trauma

Nursing Diagnoses
- Pain
- Impaired physical mobility
- Risk for fluid volume deficit

Common Complaints
- Pain

Triage Rating
- Urgent to emergent

Related Factors
- Associated with blunt force injury. In the elderly population, a low-velocity force such as a fall may result in a nondisplaced pelvic ring fracture. In young patients, high velocity forces, especially from motor vehicle crashes or falls from heights, can produce more serious pelvic fractures.

Assessment Findings
- Bruising of flank, perineal, or groin area
- Pain with compression of ischial tuberosities or over symphysis pubis
- Possible vaginal, urethral, or rectal bleeding
- Pelvic deformity
- Shortening of leg on affected side
- Possible hematuria or difficulty with voiding
- Possible hypotension
- Possible tachycardia
- Possible pale, diaphoretic skin
- Possible restlessness

Diagnostics
- Radiographic studies: pelvic films indicating area of fracture; possible urethrogram or IVP; CT scan
- CBC: normal to low hemoglobin/hematocrit; possible elevated WBC from injury
- Urinalysis: possible hematura

Interventions
- Administer oxygen 6–15 L via face mask.
- Insert IV and infuse NS fluid.
- Obtain blood samples for CBC, chemistries, type and crossmatch, PT and PTT studies.
- Insert indwelling urinary catheter if no blood at the urinary meatus.
- Administer pain relief medication:
  - **Meperidine** 25–100 mg IV/IM *or* **morphine sulfate** 2–10 mg IV.
- Monitor level of consciousness, BP, pulse rate and rhythm, pulse oximetry, respiratory rate, urinary output, and pain relief.

Disposition   Admission to operating suite, critical care area, or medical/surgical unit.

Femur Fracture

Etiology
- Trauma

Nursing Diagnoses
- Pain
- Impaired physical mobility
- Risk for fluid volume deficit
- Risk for infection
- Risk for impaired gas exchange

Common Complaints
- Pain

Triage Rating
- Urgent to emergent

Related Factors
- Associated with direct or indirect trauma. Falls in the elderly population are a common mechanism of injury. Extensive soft tissue swelling may occur with considerable blood loss. Popliteal nerves and vessels may be injured concurrently.

Assessment Findings
- Restlessness, decreasing level of consciousness if large amount of blood loss
- Pale, diaphoretic skin
- Hypotension if large volume loss
- Tachycardia
- Tachypnea
- Shortening and external rotation of affected leg
- Swelling of thigh on affected leg
- Possible visible deformity

Diagnostics
- Radiographic studies: femur film indicating area of fracture
- CBC: normal to low hemoglobin/hematocrit; possible elevated WBC from injury

Interventions
- Administer oxygen 6–15 L via face mask.
- Insert IV and infuse NS fluid.
- Obtain blood samples for CBC, chemistries, type and crossmatch, PT and PTT studies.
- Stabilize fractured leg using pillows or traction splint.
- Insert indwelling urinary catheter if no blood at the urinary meatus.
- Administer pain relief medication:
  - **Meperidine** 25–100 mg IV/IM *or* **morphine sulfate** 2–10 mg IV.
- Monitor level of consciousness, BP, pulse rate and rhythm, pulse oximetry, respiratory rate, urinary output, pain relief.

Disposition
Admission to operating suite, critical care area, or medical/surgical unit.

Thermal Burn Injury

Etiology
- Trauma, exposure to flames/smoke

Nursing Diagnoses
- Pain
- Impaired skin integrity
- Fluid volume deficit
- Altered tissue perfusion
- Risk for infection
- Risk for impaired gas exchange

Common Complaints
- Pain, possible hoarseness if concurrent smoke inhalation

Triage Rating
- Emergent

Related Factors
- Tissue damage from intense heat exposure is the result of coagulation of cellular protein and is directly related to temperature degree and length of exposure. Thermal burns that occur when the patient is in an enclosed space are often associated with smoke inhalation. Depth of burned tissue is classified as superficial, partial, or full-thickness burn.

Assessment Findings
- Restlessness, decreased level of consciousness, or coma may be associated with smoke inhalation
- Hoarseness, singed nasal hairs, blistered or reddened oral mucosa, and carbonaceous sputum are associated with smoke inhalation
- Presence of burned tissue: red, dry area without blisters (superficial); blisters (partial); white, charred, dry, or leathery tissue (full)
- Extent of burn based on Rule of Nines or Lund-Browder chart
- Hypotension if extensive partial or full-thickness burn
- Tachycardia
- Tachypnea
- Respiratory wheezing or rales if concurrent pulmonary injury from smoke

Diagnostics
- Radiographic studies: chest films possibly indicating pulmonary involvement
- Pulse oximetry: may be normal or <94%
- ABG: pH may be normal or <7.35, PaO_2 normal or <80 mm Hg, $PaCO_2$ normal to >45 mm Hg
- Carboxyhemoglobin: may be increased to 10% or higher
- CBC: normal to increased hematocrit
- Electrolytes: sodium level normal to <130 mEq; potassium normal to >5 mEq

Interventions
- Consider administration of oxygen 6–15 L via face mask or intubation if laryngeal edema develops.
- Decrease further tissue damage by removing jewelry or clothing and cooling tissue with cool NS compresses.
- Insert IV and infuse NS fluid according to fluid formula.*
- Obtain blood samples for CBC, chemistries, carboxyhemoglobin, possible type and crossmatch, PT and PTT studies.
- Administer pain relief medication: –**Meperidine** 25–100 mg increments IV *or* **morphine sulfate** 2–20 mg IV.
- Administer **dT** 0.5 mL IM if required.
- Insert indwelling urinary catheter.
- Consider insertion of nasogastric tube and attach to suction.
- Assist with nonviable tissue debridement and/or escharotomy.
- Assist with escharectomy procedure as required for circumferential burns.
- Apply burn dressing with topical antimicrobial agent if patient not being transferred to a burn center.†
- Monitor level of consciousness, BP, pulse rate and rhythm, pulse oximetry, ABG, respiratory rate, pain relief, urinary output.

*Fluid replacement formulas: based on patient weight and percent (%) of body surface area (BSA) burned. In burns that encompass >50% BSA, fluid requirements are calculated as though only 50% of the body had been burned.

Brooke Formula
- Colloid fluid: 0.5 mL/kg/% BSA burned
- Crystalloid fluid: 1.5 mL/kg/% BSA burned
- Of the total estimated fluid replacement: 1/2 is administered in the first 8 hours following the injury, 1/4 of the total in the subsequent 8 hours, and 1/4 of the total in third 8 hours of a 24-hour period

Parkland (Baxter) Formula
- Crystalloid fluid: 4 mL/kg/% BSA burned
- Administration rate is the same as the Brooke formula

†American Burn Association Guidelines for Burn Center Referral

1. Partial and full-thickness burns >10% BSA in patients <10 or >50 years of age; 20% BSA for all other age groups
2. Partial and full-thickness burns involving face, hands, feet, genitalia, perineum, major joints
3. Full-thickness burns >5% in any age group
4. Significant electrical or chemical burn injury
5. Presence of inhalation injury, concomitant trauma, or preexisting illness
6. Requirement of qualified personnel, equipment, or special social or emotional support is involved

Disposition   Admission to critical care area or transfer to regional burn center for all injuries other than minor superficial or partial-thickness burn.

Electrical Burn Injury

Etiology
- Trauma, exposure to high-voltage electricity

Nursing Diagnoses
- Altered tissue perfusion: renal
- Impaired skin integrity

Common Complaints
- Pain, may be in cardiac or respiratory arrest

Triage Rating
- Emergent

Related Factors
- Electrical current entry into body tissue causes electrical burns. Entrance and exit wounds may be the only visible injury, but extensive damage is frequently present between the wound sites. Severity of injury is dependent on intensity and type of current, contact duration, tissue resistance, and the path of the current. The majority of electrical injuries result from contact with high-voltage power sources or lines. Alternating current (AC) is more dangerous than direct current (DC) and often involves the areas of the hands and feet. The formation of ocular cataracts may occur after injury.

Assessment Findings
- Possible coma, respiratory or cardiac arrest
- Visible entrance wound: may appear dry and charred
- Visible exit wound: may have "exploded" appearance
- Tissue edema of electrical current path
- Possible cardiac dysrhythmias

Diagnostics
- ECG: may demonstrate asystole, ventricular fibrillation, or other dysrhythmias
- Cardiac enzymes: may be elevated (CK-MB) if cardiac involvement
- Urinalysis: presence of myoglobin possible
- Radiographic studies: spinal or bone films should be considered if a fall occurred or if prolonged tetany was present

Interventions
- Initiate CPR and ALS measures if required.
- Immobilize full spinal column if history of fall or tetany.
- Insert IV and infuse NS fluid.*
- Consider insertion of indwelling urinary catheter.
- Administer medication to assist with diuresis and urine alkalinization if myoglobulin is present: –**Mannitol** 0.25 g/kg IV *and* **sodium bicarbonate** IV to maintain urine pH >7.45.
- Monitor level of consciousness, BP, pulse rate and rhythm, pulse oximetry, respiratory rate, urinary output, and tissue swelling.

*IV fluids are administered at a rate to maintain an hourly urine output of 75–100 mL in an adult or 2 mL/kg in an infant or child.

Disposition   Admission to operating suite for possible fasciotomy if muscle compartment pressures are >30 mm Hg, critical care area, or transfer to regional burn center.

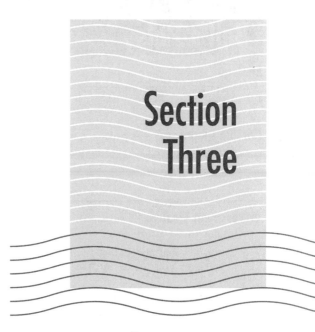

Section Three

Frequently Encountered Emergency Illness/Injuries

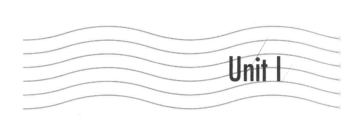

Unit I

Neurologic and Neuromuscular Conditions

Bell's Palsy

Etiology
- Unknown, possibly viral organism

Nursing Diagnoses
- Pain
- Risk for injury

Common Complaints
- Sudden onset of unilateral facial weakness/paralysis, decreased taste, difficulty swallowing, facial pain

Triage Rating
- Nonurgent

Related Factors
- The majority of cases occur in persons >40 years of age. There is facial nerve swelling with subsequent compression and ischemia. Only the seventh cranial nerve is affected.

Assessment Findings
- Eyelid lag on affected side
- Upward eyeball movement on affected side with attempt to close eye
- Widened palpebral fissure with inability to close affected eye
- Flattened nasolabial fold on affected side
- Drooping of mouth on affected side
- Drooling
- Inability to wrinkle forehead on affected side
- Possible speech difficulty

Diagnostics
- None if diagnosis is clear
- If unclear, radiographic studies: CT scan of brain

Interventions
- Explain Bell's palsy to patient.
- Administer medications:
  - **1% methylcellulose** to affected eye.
  - **Prednisone** 40–60 mg PO and for 10-day course.
- Manually close affected eyelid and apply eye patch.

Disposition   Release to home with follow-up referral to primary care physician, otolaryngologist, or neurologist.

Cerebral Vascular Accident

Etiology
- Arteriosclerotic disease, emboli, intracranial hemorrhage, hypoperfusion

Nursing Diagnoses
- Altered tissue perfusion: cerebral
- Impaired verbal communication
- Risk for ineffective airway clearance

Common Complaints
- Sudden onset of weakness, speech deficits, incontinence, altered mental status, visual disturbances

Triage Rating
- Emergent

Related Factors
- Causative factors result in a decrease or cessation of cerebral blood flow and subsequent loss of functional brain tissue. Deficits, both temporary and permanent, depend on vessel involvement, extent of damage, and amount of collateral blood flow. Associative risk factors include diabetes, congestive heart failure, atrial fibrillation, recent myocardial infarction, cardiac valvular disease, and migraine headaches. May be categorized as **transient ischemic attack** (maximal dysfunction within 5 minutes and resolution within 15 minutes), **progressing stroke** (progressive development of neurologic symptoms), and **completed stroke** (prolonged neurologic deficit lasting >21 days). Although stroke is uncommon in children, it can occur. It is frequently associated with congenital heart disease and most commonly occurs between the ages of 1 and 5 years.

Assessment Findings
- Carotid circulation deficit:
  - Restlessness, decreasing level of consciousness
  - Speech deficits of expressive or receptive dysphasia
  - Visual deficits of ipsilateral temporary blindness or contralateral loss of sight in the lateral halves of the eyes
  - Contralateral hemiparesis or hemiplegia
- Vertebral basilar deficit:
  - Restlessness or decreasing level of consciousness
  - Speech deficits of dysphonia, dysarthria
  - Dysphagia
  - Visual deficits of cortical blindness, field deficits, or diplopia
  - Motor weakness in more than one limb
- Possible hypertension
- Incontinence

Diagnostics
- Radiographic studies: CT scan, possible Doppler flow studies
- ECG: may indicate presence of atrial fibrillation or other cardiac dysrhythmias
- PT and PTT studies: baseline coagulation study especially if anticoagulant therapy is involved
- Possible lumbar puncture after CT scan

Interventions
- Administer oxygen 6–15 L via face mask or bag-valve-mask device.
- Assist with possible intubation and mechanical ventilation.
- Position patient with head midline.
- Insert IV or saline lock.
- Obtain blood samples for PT, PTT, CBC, chemistries.
- Insert nasogastric tube and attach to suction.
- Insert indwelling urinary catheter.
- Administer medications to improve cerebral blood flow:
  - **Nimodipine** 60 mg PO (if subarachnoid hemorrhage).
  - **Mannitol** 1–2 g/kg IV infusion of 20% solution over 5–10 minutes.
  - **Heparin** IV if no intracranial bleeding is present.
  - **Antithrombolytic** medications according to institution protocol.
- Monitor level of consciousness, BP, pulse rate and rhythm, pulse oximetry, respiratory rate, urinary output.

Disposition   Admission to critical care area.

Chronic Headache

Etiology
- May be related to stress, precipitating events, or unknown causes

Nursing Diagnoses
- Pain

Common Complaints
- Headache, nausea, vomiting, photophobia, muscle spasms
  - **Tension headache**: pain frequently gradual in onset; located bilaterally in occipital or frontal lobes; described as pressure or a tight band of pain that is constant, nonthrobbing
  - **Migraine headache**: frequently preceded by an aura; often hemicranial but may be bilateral; described as throbbing

Triage Rating
- Nonurgent to urgent

Related Factors
- Precipitating events may include ingestion of certain foods or wine, menses, stress, and vasodilator medications or oral contraceptives. With migraine-type headaches, an aura of visual disturbances is common.

Assessment Findings
- Absence of focal neurologic deficits
- Pale skin color
- Eye pain with the presence of light
- Emesis
- Possible easing of pain when the ipsilateral carotid or superficial temporal artery is compressed

Diagnostics
- Usually none
- Radiographic studies: CT scan of brain if pain is described as "worst headache pain in life" or if different from usual headache pain

Interventions
- Place patient in a darkened room.
- Administer pain relieving medications:
  –**Meperidine** 50–150 mg IM *or* **dihydroergotamine (DHE) 45** 0.5–1 mg IV *or* **sumatriptan** 6 mg SC.
- Administer antiemetic medications:
  –**Metoclopramide** 10 mg IV *or* **promethazine** 25 mg IV/IM *or* **prochlorperazine** 10 mg IV/IM *or* **hydralazine** 25–50 mg IM.
- Monitor pain relief.

Disposition   Release to home.

Concussion

Etiology
- Trauma

Nursing Diagnoses
- Altered tissue perfusion: cerebral
- Pain

Common Complaints
- Possible loss of consciousness, amnesia (retrograde or posttraumatic), headache, vomiting, sleepiness

Triage Rating
- Nonurgent to urgent

Related Factors
- Results from either a direct forceful blow to the skull or acceleration/deceleration forces. If a documented loss of consciousness lasted for >5 minutes, consider hospitalization.

Assessment Findings
- Alert or possible disorientation surrounding memory of injury event
- Nonprojectile vomiting
- No focal neurologic findings

Diagnostics
- Radiographic studies: CT of brain if documented loss of consciousness

Interventions
- Monitor for improving level of consciousness, BP, pulse rate and rhythm, respiratory rate, pupil reactions.

Disposition   Majority of patients are discharged to home with appropriate instructions for postconcussion syndrome.

Guillian-Barré Syndrome

Etiology
- Unknown

Nursing Diagnoses
- Risk for ineffective breathing patterns
- Impaired physical mobility

Common Complaints
- Sensory numbness or paresthesia in a stocking-glove pattern, muscle pain or tenderness, symmetric ascending muscle weakness

Triage Rating
- Urgent

Related Factors
- Symptoms often follow viral illness, immunizations—especially influenza, mild upper respiratory illness, or gastroenteritis. Affects all age groups but children often encounter a milder case.

Assessment Findings
- Numbness or paresthesia of hands and feet
- Muscle weakness of the lower extremities
- Decreased or absent reflexes even in muscles not yet demonstrating weakness
- Weakness of respiratory muscles
- Cranial nerve involvement especially CN VII
- Possible hypertension
- Possible tachycardia

Diagnostics
- Lumbar puncture: elevated protein (100–400 mg/dl) in CSF

Interventions
- Support respiratory effort: may require intubation and mechanical ventilation.
- Insert IV or saline lock.
- Position patient with slight elevation of the head of the bed.
- Insert nasogastric tube and attach to suction.
- Insert indwelling or intermittent urinary catheter.
- Monitor respiratory rate, BP, pulse rate and rhythm, pulse oximetry, urinary output.

Disposition   Admission to critical care area.

Meningitis

Etiology
- Bacterial, viral, fungal organisms

Nursing Diagnoses
- Infection
- Pain
- Altered tissue perfusion: cerebral

Common Complaints
- Fever, headache, neck stiffness, vomiting, irritability

Triage Rating
- Urgent to emergent

Related Factors
- Both adult and pediatric age groups may be affected. The incidence of bacterial infections is highest in children under the age of 1 year. The most common causing organisms include *Haemophilus influenzae*, *Streptococcus pneumoniae*, and *Neisseria meningitidis*. Infants may demonstrate only symptoms of vomiting, lethargy, irritability, or fever.

Assessment Findings
- Alert, irritable, or decreased level of consciousness
- Increased temperature
- Photophobia
- Meningeal irritation findings:
  - Meningimus
  - Positive Kernig's sign
  - Positive Brudzinski's sign
- Petechial rash may be present
- Possible bulging fontanelle in infants

Diagnostics
- CBC: elevated WBC with bacterial cause, normal to low WBC in viral cause
- Blood cultures
- Serum glucose: may be decreased in infants <6 months
- Serum chemistries: presence of hyponatremia possible
- PT and PTT studies: presence of clotting abnormalities possible
- Lumbar puncture: normal to increased opening pressure
  - *Bacterial cause*:
    - WBC 2000–20,000 µ/L
    - Decreased glucose
    - Elevated protein
    - Gram's stain: bacteria
  - *Viral cause*:
    - WBC <500 µ/L
    - Normal glucose
    - Normal protein
    - Gram's stain: no bacteria
- Radiographic studies: chest

Interventions
- Administer oxygen 6–15 L via face mask.
- Insert IV and infuse NS fluid.
- Obtain blood samples for CBC, chemistries, coagulation studies, cultures.
- Administer antibiotic medications:*
  - **Penicillin G** 20–24 million units/d IV infusion (Peds: 250,000 µ/kg/d) *or* **ampicillin** 1–2 g IV infusion (Peds: 100–200 mg/kg) *or* **chloramphenicol** 1 g IV infusion (Peds: 50–100 mg/kg/d) *or* **cefuroxine** 1.5–3 g IV infusion (Peds: 200–240 mg/kg/d) *or* **gentamicin** 3–5 g IV infusion (Peds: 6–7.5 mg/kg/d) or combinations of antibiotics.
  - **Ceftizoxime** 1–2 g IV infusion (Peds: 50 mg/kg) *or* **ceftriaxone** 1–2 g IV infusion (Peds: 100 mg/kg/d).
- Administer antipyretic medication:
  - **Acetaminophen** 10 mg/kg PO, PR.
- Administer pain relief medication:
  - **Meperidine** 50–100 mg IM/IV.
- Consider insertion of nasogastric tube and attach to suction.
- Consider insertion of indwelling urinary catheter.
- Monitor level of consciousness, BP, pulse rate and rhythm, pulse oximetry, respiratory rate, temperature, pain relief, urinary output.

*Consider administering prophylatic **rifampin** 10–20 mg/kg up to 600 mg PO to close family members or contacts if the patient is diagnosed with meningococcal *(Neisseria)* meningitis.

Disposition   Patients with diagnosed bacterial meningitis require hospitalization. Patients with viral meningitis may be released to home with close follow-up.

Myasthenia Gravis (MG)

Etiology
- Immunologic disorder

Nursing Diagnoses
- Risk for ineffective breathing pattern
- Sensory/perceptual alteration

Common Complaints
- Weakness, hoarseness, voice quality changes, double vision, eyelid lag

Triage Rating
- Urgent

Related Factors
- Symptoms have often been present for a long time before a diagnosis of MG because symptoms are intermittent. Rest periods appear to improve strength. The course of the disease is variable, with fatalities most common during the first year of the disease. Congenital MG should be suspected in infants with bilateral ptosis.

Assessment Findings
- Possible respiratory difficulty
- Fatigue
- Facial contractures
- Nasal voice quality
- Ability to manually open patient's jaw
- Asymmetric weakness of CN III, IV, or VI resulting in ptosis and diplopia
- Tendon reflexes: normal
- Cholinergic crisis symptoms:
  - Bradycardia
  - Sweating
  - Salivation
  - Diarrhea
  - Hypotension

Diagnostics
- Improvement in cranial nerve function with the administration of edrophonium chloride

Interventions
- Administer oxygen 6–15 L via face mask if respiratory difficulty is present.
- Prepare for intubation and mechanical ventilation if cholinergic crisis is present.
- Insert IV or saline lock.
- Administer diagnostic medication:
  - **Edrophonium** 2 mg IV over 30 seconds. If no improvement, administer an additional 8 mg.
- Administer anticholinergic medication if crisis is present:
  - **Atropine** dose titrated to maintain heart rate above 50 bpm.
- Monitor respiratory rate, pulse oximetry, cardiac rhythm, pulse rate and rhythm, BP, muscle strength.

Disposition
Patients in cholinergic crisis require hospitalization for supportive care. Patients without respiratory symptoms may be released to home with close follow-up.

Seizure

Etiology
- Seizure disorder, fever, drug intoxication/withdrawal, trauma, metabolic disorders, pregnancy, CVA

Nursing Diagnoses
- Altered tissue perfusion: cerebral
- Risk for injury
- Noncompliance

Common Complaints
- Possible aura preceding seizure, tremors

Triage Rating
- Urgent to emergent

Related Factors
- Results from an underlying condition. A generalized seizure producing repetitive tonic-clonic movements is a grand mal seizure. This is followed by a postictal state, which may last from minutes to hours. Status epilepticus is multiple seizure activity without a sufficient postictal recovery period between seizures.

Assessment Findings
- Decreased or absent respirations
- Either tonic-clonic seizure activity or postictal behavior
- Possible cyanosis
- Incontinence
- Possible increased temperature

Diagnostics
- Serum chemistry–possible results: sodium <135 mEq; glucose >120 mg/dl, <45 mg/dl or normal
- CBC: possible elevation of WBC if infection present
- Anticonvulsant medication level: may be subtherapeutic or toxic
- Toxicology screen: presence of toxic substances
- Alcohol: level may range between 0 mg/dl– >500 mg/dl
- Radiographic studies: CT brain scan, chest film for possible infection, or aspiration findings
- Possible lumbar puncture

Interventions
- Position patient on left side if possible.
- Protect airway by loosening tight clothing around the neck, suction airway.
- Administer oxygen 6–15 L via face mask or bag-valve-mask device.
- Insert IV or saline lock.
- Obtain blood samples for CBC, cultures, chemistries, medication levels, toxicology.
- Administer antipyretic medication if fever present:
  –**Acetaminophen** 15 mg/kg PR.
- Administer antiseizure medications:
  –**Diazepam** 5–10 mg IV if seizure activity is present.
  –**Phenytoin** 1 g IV or PO (if IV mix only with NS solution and infuse at rate 50 mg/min or less).
- Administer other medications depending on cause as needed.*
- Undress child if fever is precipitating cause.
- Monitor seizure activity, pulse rate and rhythm, BP, pulse oximetry.

*Medications depending on cause:
- Pregnancy-induced hypertension with seizure: **magnesium sulfate** 1–2 g IM, IV
- Infection: antibiotic medication depending on causative organism (PO, IM, IV)
- Alcohol-induced: **magnesium** 2 g, **multivitamins, thiamine** 100 mg IV infusion
  For tremors, **lorazepam** 0. 5–2 mg PO, IV
  For withdrawal, **chlordiazepoxide** 25–100 mg IM, IV

Disposition   If seizure activity is terminated and the cause of the seizure is identified and treatable, the patient may be released to home. If cause is undetermined, or seizure activity is not controlled, hospitalization is required.

Trigeminal Neuralgia

Etiology
• Unknown

Nursing Diagnoses
• Pain

Common Complaints
• Paroxysmal excruciating pain in jaw

Triage Rating
• Nonurgent

Related Factors
• Inflammation of the fifth cranial nerve produces pain over the affected area. Trigger points may be present and will reproduce the pain when touched. Other stimulants that may reproduce pain include cold, wind, talking, and chewing. The condition is more common in women, especially over the age of 40 years.

Assessment Findings
• Trigger point pain reproduction
• Drooping of corner of mouth on affected side

Diagnostics
• None

Interventions
• Administer medications to relieve pain:
  –**Phenytoin** 250 mg IV (may diminish the acute episode).
  –**Carbamazepine** 200–600 mg PO *or* **baclofen** 5–20 mg PO.
  –Narcotic medications are usually not effective.
• Assist with trigeminal nerve block.
• Monitor pain relief, BP, pulse rate and rhythm.

Disposition   Once pain has been controlled, the majority of patients can be released to home and with outpatient treatment.

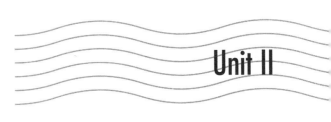

Unit II

Ocular Conditions

Central Retinal Artery Occlusion

Etiology
- Thrombus, emboli, orbital hematomas, acute angle closure glaucoma

Nursing Diagnoses
- Altered tissue perfusion: optic

Common Complaints
- Sudden loss of vision (usually unilateral)

Triage Rating
- Emergent

Related Factors
- With occlusion of the retinal artery, blood flow to the retina is diminished. Receptors in the retina begin to degenerate within 30 to 60 minutes. Recovery is usually minimal. Risk-related factors include hypertension, diabetes, arteriosclerotic or cardiovascular disease, and sickle cell anemia. The hallmark sign associated with this problem is the absence of pain.

Assessment Findings
- Diminished visual acuity
- Fundoscopic findings:
  - Pale optic disk
  - Macular edema
  - Cherry-red fovea
  - Narrowed arteries
  - Dilated and nonreactive pupil

Diagnostics
- Ocular pressure measurement: may be increased
- Visual acuity: decreased in affected eye

Interventions
- Physician performs digital globe massage.
- Instruct patient to breathe into a paper bag to rebreathe carbon dioxide.
- Insert IV or saline lock.
- Administer medications to lower intraocular pressure:
  - **Acetazolamide** 250 mg IV.
  - **Mannitol 20%** 300 mL IV over 20 minutes.
  - **Timolol** 1 drop in affected eye.
- Administer medications to improve optic blood flow:
  - **Heparin** 10,000 units IV.
  - **Nitroglycerin** 0.4 mg SL.
- Assist with immediate ophthalmologic referral for possible surgical decompression of anterior chamber.

Disposition   Hospitalization for further treatment by an ophthalmologist.

Conjunctivitis

Etiology
- Viral or bacterial organisms, chemicals, allergy

Nursing Diagnoses
- Pain
- Risk for infection

Common Complaints
- Pain, eye itching, eye discharge, matted eyelashes

Triage Rating
- Nonurgent

Related Factors
- Conjunctivitis of an infectious cause is often associated with an upper respiratory infection. It is most common in school-aged children and is highly contagious. The most common causing bacterial organisms include *Streptococcus*, *Staphylococcus*, *Pneumococcus*, and *Gonococcus*. Conjuctivitis caused by *Chlamydia* can lead to corneal scarring and blindness if left untreated. Other considerations of conjunctivitis include infestation of crab louse, or systemic infections such as rubeola, rubella, and Kawasaki syndrome.

Assessment Findings
- Conjunctival injection
- Possible enlarged preauricular lymph nodes
- Crusting discharge at medial canthus
- Itching of eyes
- Normal visual acuity
- If allergy related: possible respiratory wheezes

Diagnostics
- Visual acuity: normal
- Slit lamp examination: no ciliary flush, no cells or flare in anterior chamber
- Fluorescein staining for evidence of corneal abrasion

Interventions
- Instill antibiotic eyedrops:
  - **Sulfacetamide** 1–3 drops, or ointment* *or* **gentamicin** 1–3 drops or ointment.*
- If allergic conjunctivitis administer:
  - **Diphenhydramine** 25–50 mg PO.

*Use ophthalmic eye ointment in infants and toddlers.

Other antibiotic medications depending on identified cause include:

- Oral **trimethoprim-sulfamethoxazole** or a**moxicillin-clavulanate** if associated with otitis media.
- Oral **doxycycline** if associated with *Chlamydia* organisims, along with **erythromycin** ophthalmic ointment. In adults sexual partner also requires treatment.

Disposition
Release to home. Provide instructions concerning careful handwashing, use of individual linens, and eye medications.

Corneal Abrasion

Etiology
- Entrance of foreign object into cornea, exposure to ultraviolet light, contact lenses, infection

Nursing Diagnoses
- Pain
- Risk for infection

Common Complaints
- Pain, excessive tearing, gritty feeling in eye

Triage Rating
- Urgent

Related Factors
- One of the most common eye problems encountered in the ED. Metallic objects in the eye can leave a rust ring, which must be removed as soon as possible.

Assessment Findings
- Excessive tearing from affected eye
- Photophobia
- Conjunctival edema and erythema
- Possible visible foreign object in affected eye
- Ulceration with abrasion from contact lens appears as white or opaque with ill-defined margins

Diagnostics
- Visual acuity: normal to decreased
- Eversion of eyelids: may reveal identifiable foreign object
- Fluorescein stain: identifiable stin uptake on affected cornea with ultraviolet light or with slit lamp examination; possible presence of punctate lesions

Interventions
- Instill topical anesthetic medication:
  - **Proparacaine** 2 drops in affected eye.
- Remove obvious foreign object using irrigation or 18-gauge needle.
- Assist with or perform fluorescein stain procedure.
- Remove rust ring with Optha-Burr.
- Administer antibiotic medication as required:
  - **Sulfacetamide** 1–3 drops or ointment to affected eye *or* **gentamicin** 1–3 drops or ointment to affected eye.
- Administer **dT** 0.5 mL IM if >5 years since booster.
- Consider patching affected eye.*

*Eye patching is currently controversial. If the corneal abrasion is caused by contact lenses, *eye patching is absolutely contraindicated* because of the possible presence of *Pseudomonas* organisms and the potential for further corneal injury.

Disposition   Release to home with follow-up referral within 24 hours. Systemic pain relief medication such as **acetaminophen with codeine** or **hydrocodone** must be prescribed for the patient.

Glaucoma

Etiology
- Obstruction or narrowing of Schlemm's canal

Nursing Diagnoses
- Pain
- Altered tissue perfusion: optic
- Sensory/perceptual alteration: visual

Common Complaints
- Pain, decreased vision, nausea, headache

Triage Rating
- Urgent to emergent

Related Factors
- The ocular ciliary body continues to produce aqueous humor at a normal rate, but uptake of fluid is impeded. Intraocular pressure increases with resulting compression of optic structures. The disease may be chronic or acute. Visual disturbances such as blurred vision and seeing halos surrounding single light sources are not symptoms of open-angle glaucoma, as commonly believed.

Assessment Findings
- Hazy, steamy appearing cornea
- Reddened conjunctiva
- Decreased visual acuity
- Semidilated, nonreactive pupil
- Fundoscopic findings:
  - Increased cup/disk ratio
  - Shallow anterior chamber
- Emesis
- Photophobia

Diagnostics
- Visual acuity: decreased
- Tonometry: intraocular pressure reading above 20 mm Hg

Interventions
- Instill medications to decrease intraocular pressure:
  - **Pilocarpine** 1–4% 1–2 drops to affected eye q5min × 3 and possibly to unaffected eye.
- Insert IV or saline lock.
- Administer medications to decrease intraocular fluid:
  - **Mannitol 20%** 250–500 mL IV over 2–3 hours.
  - **Acetazolamide** 500 mg PO or 250 mg IV.
- Administer medications to decrease emesis.
- Administer medications to relieve pain.
- Monitor intraocular pressure, BP, pulse rate and rhythm, pain relief.

Disposition   Further evaluation by an ophthalmologist on an immediate outpatient basis or through hospitalization is required.

Hyphema

Etiology
- Trauma

Nursing Diagnoses
- Sensory/perceptual alteration: visual

Common Complaints
- Possible pain and blurring of vision

Triage Rating
- Urgent to emergent

Related Factors
- Blunt forces to the head or eyes may cause bleeding from the vascular iris and ciliary body. This bleeding fills the anterior chamber, often resulting in a half-moon-shaped hyphema. Episodes of rebleeding may occur within 3–5 days of the original bleeding. Patients with a history of sickle-cell disease have a greater risk of developing a hyphema without an associated history of injury. Glaucoma may be a long-term complication of hyphema.

Assessment Findings
- Visible blood in the anterior chamber: remains horizontal in spite of body position changes
- Blurring of vision without change in visual acuity

Diagnostics
- Visual acuity: may be normal
- Slit lamp examination: visible blood in the anterior chamber
- Tonometry: intraocular pressures may be increased above 20 mm Hg
- Radiographic studies: CT of ocular orbits

Interventions
- Position patient with head of bed elevated to 30–45 degrees.
- Patch affected eye with metal shield and consider patching unaffected eye.
- Monitor hyphema level, BP, pulse rate and rhythm.

Disposition Referral to an ophthalmologist is mandatory, and hospitalization may be required.

Other Avoid administering aspirin or aspirin-containing medications for pain relief. Advise patient that the wearing of protective eye gear is the best prevention against sustaining subsequent eye injuries.

Iritis/Uveitis

Etiology
- Trauma or associated with rheumatic disease, syphilis, ankylosing spondylitis, tuberculosis, HIV

Nursing Diagnoses
- Pain
- Sensory/perceptual alteration: visual

Common Complaints
- Moderate to severe unilateral eye pain, decreased visual acuity, photophobia, nausea/vomiting

Triage Rating
- Urgent to emergent

Related Factors
- Iritis/uveitis is more common in adults, with men being affected twice as often as women. Complications include glaucoma, band keratopathy, and cataracts.

Assessment Findings
- Small, irregular pupil on affected side with slowed reaction
- Upper eyelid edema
- Reddened conjunctiva/sclera
- Ciliary flush
- Consensual photophobia
- Fundoscopic findings:
  - Cloudy vitreous
  - Retinal patches

Diagnostics
- Visual acuity: decreased
- Tonometry: normal intraocular pressure <20 mm Hg
- Slit lamp examination: cornea clear, cells and flare in anterior chamber

Interventions
- Place patient in darkened room environment.
- Administer cycloplegic eyedrops to affected eye:
  - **Cyclopentolate (Cyclogyl)** drops.
- Monitor pain relief, BP, pulse rate and rhythm.

Disposition   Referral to an ophthalmologist within 24 hours for continued outpatient treatment.

Ocular Chemical Exposure

Etiology
- Trauma

Nursing Diagnoses
- Pain
- Sensory/perception alteration: visual

Common Complaints
- Pain, decreased vision

Triage Rating
- Urgent to emergent

Related Factors
- Chemical bases are usually either acidic or alkalotic. The alkaline substances can cause a coagulation necrosis as well as progressive ocular damage.

Assessment Findings
- Excessive tearing in affected eye(s)
- Decreased visual acuity
- Possible corneal whitening
- Conjunctival edema and infection
- Redness and edema of eyelids

Diagnostics
- Visual acuity: decreased in affected eye(s)
- Fluorescein staining: possible stain uptake on cornea visible with ultraviolet light or slit lamp examination

Interventions
- Administer anesthetic medication:
  –**Proparacaine** 2 drops in affected eye.
- Irrigate affected eye with copious amounts of NS.
- Administer antibiotic medication as required:
  –**Sulfacetamide** 1–3 drops or ointment to affected eye *or* **gentamicin** 1–3 drops or ointment to affected eye.
- If corneal abrasion present administer:
  –**dT** 0.5 mL IM if necessary.
- Monitor pain relief and visual acuity changes.

Disposition   Provide referral to an ophthalmologist for further treatment on an outpatient basis. Patching the affected eye is currently controversial.

Ocular Globe Rupture

Etiology
• Trauma

Nursing Diagnoses
• Pain
• Sensory/perceptual alteration: visual

Common Complaints
• Pain, decreased visual acuity

Triage Rating
• Emergent

Related Factors
• Either penetrating or blunt forces directed at the eye may cause a globe rupture. If a penetrating object is still in place, it should not be removed in the ED.

Assessment Findings
• Shallow-appearing anterior chamber
• Ocular hemorrhage
• Pupil irregularity
• Decreased visual acuity

Diagnostics
• Visual acuity: decreased
• Radiographic studies: CT scan of ocular orbits and intraocular structures may demonstrate imbedded foreign object

Interventions
• Patch affected eye with metal shield.
• Insert IV or saline lock.
• Administer pain relief medication:
  –**Meperidine** 25–100 mg IV/IM *or* **morphine sulfate** 2–10 mg titrated to pain relief.
• Administer antibiotic medication.
• Administer **dT** 0.5 mL IM as needed.
• Monitor BP, pulse rate and rhythm, respiratory rate, pain relief.

Disposition   Admit to operating suite for repair or enucleation.

Orbital/Periorbital Cellulitis

Etiology
- Bacterial or fungal organisms, trauma

Nursing Diagnoses
- Pain

Common Complaints
- Fever, pain in and around the eye, change in visual acuity

Triage Rating
- Urgent

Related Factors
- Commonly caused by *Streptococcus pneumoniae, Staphylococcus aureus,* or *Haemophilus influenzae* in children. In patients with diabetes, fungi may be the precipitating cause. The organism frequently enters the orbit via the paranasal sinus. The infection may spread to the meninges or cavernous sinus.

Assessment Findings
- Edema and erythema of eyelids and periorbital tissue
- Exophthalmos (or proptosis) of affected eye if globe affected
- Conjunctival edema
- Fundoscopic findings:
  - Blurred disk margins
- Limited eye movements in all fields

Diagnostics
- Visual acuity: decreased
- Radiographic studies: plain or CT scan of sinus may reveal evidence of sinusitis
- CBC: WBC elevated because of infection

Interventions
- Insert IV or saline lock.
- Obtain laboratory studies of CBC, blood culture, and possibly periorbital tissue fluid.
- Administer antibiotic medication:
  - **Cefuroxime** 750 mg–1.5 g IV infusion (Peds: 75–150 mg/k/d).

Disposition   Hospitalization is mandatory for any patient with orbital cellulitis. Patients with periorbital cellulitis may be treated on an outpatient basis after receiving an IV or IM dose of antibiotics with follow-up within 24 hours.

Retinal Detachment

Etiology
- Trauma or history of related factors

Nursing Diagnoses
- Sensory/perceptual alteration: visual

Common Complaints
- Visual changes of seeing flashing lights, visual field loss, cloudy vision

Triage Rating
- Urgent

Related Factors
- Patients with a history of retinal detachment, previous ocular surgery, intraocular tumors, renal failure, or ocular inflammatory disease are at an increased risk for retinal detachment. Blunt force injury to the face or head may also produce retinal detachment. Additionally, persons over the age of 60 are at an increased risk. The onset may be sudden or gradual; if neglected, blindness may result. As the sensory retina separates from the underlying epithelium, fluid begins to accumulate between the two structures.

Assessment Findings
- Diminished visual fields
- Fundoscopic findings through dilated pupil:
  - Grayish-blue retinal membrane that folds or balloons out

Diagnostics
- Visual acuity: decreased
- Tonometry: low to normal intraocular pressure readings <20 mm Hg

Interventions
- Assist patient into the supine position.
- Patch both eyes.

Disposition   Obtain immediate ophthalmologist referral and hospitalize patient for evaluation of surgical reattachment.

Subconjunctival Hemorrhage

Etiology
- Trauma, vomiting, coughing

Nursing Diagnoses
- Fear

Common Complaints
- Pain if associated with injury, noticeable blood in affected eye

Triage Rating
- Nonurgent

Related Factors
- Rupture of the conjunctival blood vessels can occur following direct injury to the eye, face, or head. Abrupt increases in intraocular pressure from coughing, sneezing, or vomiting can also cause rupture of the blood vessels.

Assessment Findings
- Blood in superficial conjunctiva
- Normal visual acuity
- Chemosis

Diagnostics
- Visual acuity: normal

Interventions
- None.

Disposition   Release to home. Further treatment can be provided on an outpatient basis. If no other injuries are present, the hemorrhage will resolve within 2 weeks.

Unit III

Ear-Nose-Throat
Conditions

Labyrinthitis

Etiology
- Bacterial or viral organism

Nursing Diagnoses
- Sensory/perceptual alteration: auditory
- Risk for fluid volume deficit

Common Complaints
- Disabling vertigo, nausea, vomiting, occasional tinnitus, possible hearing loss

Triage Rating
- Urgent

Related Factors
- More common in adults and may follow an upper respiratory infection. It may also be caused by tertiary syphilis.

Assessment Findings
- Nystagmus
- Ataxia
- Intact cranial nerve and cerebellar function
- Tachycardia
- Vomiting or dizziness with position changes
- Nylen-Barany (Dix-Hallpike) maneuver: positive for peripheral vertigo*

Diagnostics
- Serum chemistry: sodium and potassium possibly low because of vomiting
- Thyroid profile: normal
- VDRL
- Radiographic studies: possible CT scan of the brain

Interventions
- Assist patient into the supine position.
- Insert IV and infuse NS fluid.
- Obtain blood samples for chemistries and other tests.
- Administer medications to control dizziness:
  –**Meclizine** 25 mg PO.
- Administer medications to control vomiting:
  –**Prochlorperazine** 10 mg IV/IM, PR
  –**Promethazine** 25 mg IV/IM PR.
- Monitor vertigo, vomiting, BP, pulse rate and rhythm.

*Nylen-Barany (Dix-Hallpike) maneuver can differentiate a central from a peripheral vestibulopathy. To perform the maneuver, have the patient sit on the edge of the bed, then suddenly recline with the patient's head hanging 45 degrees backward and rotated 45 degrees to one side. Repeat the test two more times, first with the head rotated 45 degrees to the other side, and second with the head midline. Keep the patient's eyes open and observe for (1) vertigo and (2) time of onset of vertigo. Central vestibulopathy produces immediate mild vertigo with no lessening of signs with test repetition. Peripheral vestibulopathy produces severe vertigo in a 3- to 10-second onset and a lessening of signs with test repetition.

Disposition   Release to home if vertigo and vomiting are controlled in the ED. If symptoms are not controlled, hospitalization may be required for IV fluid replacement.

Meniere's Disease

Etiology
• Unknown

Nursing Diagnosis
• Sensory/perceptual alteration: auditory

Common Complaints
• Decreased hearing, tinnitus, episodic vertigo, nausea, vomiting

Triage Rating
• Urgent

Related Factors
• Affects persons between the ages of 40–50 years. The onset is usually gradual with a prodrome of aural fullness or pressure. Acute exacerbations occur.

Assessment Findings
• Lateral gaze nystagmus
• Pale, diaphoretic skin
• Disequilibrium: falls toward affected ear
• Intact cranial nerve function
• Nylen-Barany (Dix-Hallpike) maneuver: positive for peripheral vertigo*

Diagnostics
• Serum chemistry: sodium and potassium levels possibly low if prolonged vomiting has occurred
• Radiographic studies: possible CT scan of the brain

Interventions
• Assist patient into the supine position.
• Insert IV and infuse NS fluid.
• Obtain blood samples for CBC chemistries, and other studies.
• Administer medications to reduce vertigo:
  –**Meclizine** 25 mg PO.
• Administer medications to reduce vomiting:
  –**Prochlorperazine** 5–10 mg IV/IM, PR.
  –**Promethazine** 25 mg IV/IM, PR.

*Nylen-Barany (Dix-Hallpike) maneuver can differentiate a central from a peripheral vestibulopathy. To perform the maneuver, have the patient sit on the edge of the bed, then recline suddenly with the patient's head hanging 45 degrees backward and rotated 45 degrees to one side. Repeat the test two more times, first with the head rotated 45 degrees to the other side, and second with the head midline. Keep the patient's eyes open and observe for (1) vertigo and (2) time of onset of vertigo. Central vestibulopathy produces immediate mild vertigo with no lessening of signs with test repetition. Peripheral vestibulopathy produces severe vertigo in a 3- to 10-second onset and a lessening of signs with test repetition.

Disposition   Release to home if vertigo and vomiting are not controlled in the ED. If symptoms are controlled, hospitalization may be required for fluid replacement.

Otitis Externa

Etiology
- Frequent exposure of ear canal to water, trauma

Nursing Diagnoses
- Pain
- Infection

Common Complaints
- Ear pain

Triage Rating
- Nonurgent

Related Factors
- *Pseudomonas aeruginosa* is the primary organism, although fungi may also be a precipitating agent. All age groups may be affected. Cleaning of the ear canal with cotton swabs is also a frequent cause of infection. Persons with diabetes are at risk for developing malignant otitis externa, a serious disorder.

Assessment Findings
- Tragal tenderness
- Pain with movement of ear auricle
- Erythema and edema of auditory canal
- Possible discharge from canal
- Possible preauricular or postauricular adenopathy

Diagnostics
- None

Interventions
- Administer antibiotic medications:
  –**Polymyxin B sulfate (Cortisporin*)** otic suspension/solution 3–4 drops in canal: may require use of ear wick.
  Cefaclor *or* **amoxicillin-clavulanate** PO for severe cases.
- Administer pain relief medication:
  –**Acetaminophen with codeine** *or* **hydrocodone** PO.

***Polymyxin B sulfate (Cortisporin)** suspension should be used if unable to visualize the tympanic membrane. If the tympanic membrane is visible and intact, the solution can be used.

Disposition
Release to home. Instruct patient to keep ear canal dry and discourage the use of cotton swabs or sharp instruments to clean ears. If the patient has been treated with systemic antibiotics, follow-up should occur within 24 hours, otherwise follow-up care is in 7 days. Malignant otitis externa is a finding in the diabetic patient and requires hospitalization with aggressive treatment.

Otic Foreign Object

Etiology
- Intentional or unintentional insertion of foreign object into auditory canal

Nursing Diagnoses
- Pain
- Risk for infection

Common Complaints
- Pain, decreased hearing, possible discharge from affected ear

Triage Rating
- Nonurgent

Related Factors
- Children may attempt to place almost any object into the external auditory canal. Adults are more likely to have inserted an object to clean the canal. Insects may also have entered the canal. Removal can be difficult with as many as 10% of the objects not being successfully removed in the ED. Otitis externa is common following object removal.

Assessment Findings
- Edema and erythema of ear canal
- Visible object in canal
- Possible discharge and odor from affected ear

Diagnostics
- None

Interventions
- Remove object using alligator forceps, suction, or irrigation with room temperature water if TM intact and object is not vegetable material.
- Insect removal: kill insect first by inserting **mineral oil** or **lidocaine (Xylocaine)** into ear canal.
- Following removal, if otitis externa is present, adminster: **Polymyxin B sulfate (Cortisporin)** otic suspension/solution drops.

Disposition Release to home if object was removed in ED. If removal is not successful, refer to ear, nose, and throat specialist for possible hospitalization and surgical removal.

Otitis Media

Etiology
- Bacterial or viral organism

Nursing Diagnoses
- Pain
- Infection

Common Complaints
- Ear pain, fever; in children, crying and pulling at ears

Triage Rating
- Nonurgent

Related Factors
- Common pathogens include *Streptococcus pneumoniae*, *Haemophilus influenzae*, *Moraxella catarrhalis*, and viruses. Any condition that causes eustachian tube edema or congestion can lead to a middle ear infection. The most common age group is children <5 years of age, but can occur at any age. Contributing factors include infants who are bottle fed (especially if the bottle is propped) and households in which smoking occurs.

Assessment Findings
- Increased temperature
- Possible decrease in hearing
- Otoscope findings:
  - Full or bulging TM: possible presence of erythema
  - Absence of landmarks and distorted light reflex
  - Decreased TM motility
  - Bleb or vesicle on TM with bullous myringitis
  - Possible preauricular or postauricular or cervical lymphadenopathy

Diagnostics
- None

Interventions
- Administer antibiotic medication:
  - **Amoxicillin** 125–500 mg PO or other antibiotics depending on previous infections or allergies.
- Administer pain medications:
  - **Acetaminophen** *or* **acetaminophen with codeine** PO.
  - **Antipyrine**, **benzocaine**, *and* **oxyquinoline (Auralgan)** otic solution.

Disposition   Release to home with follow-up in 10 days.

Ruptured Tympanic Membrane

Etiology
- Untreated otitis media, barotrauma, or trauma to ear or face

Nursing Diagnoses
- Pain
- Sensory/perceptual alteration: auditory

Common Complaints
- Sudden decreased hearing, tinnitus

Triage Rating
- Nonurgent

Related Factors
- Perforations of the TM can be either central or marginal. Perforations caused by untreated infections are the most frequent cause of permanent perforations.

Assessment Findings
- Possible discharge from affected ear
- Otoscope findings: tear or perforation of TM

Diagnostics
- None

Interventions
- Administer medications:
  - **Polymyxin B sulfate (Cortisporin)** otic suspension 3–4 drops in affected ear.
  - **Amoxicillin** 125–500 mg PO.
  - **Acetaminophen with codeine** *or* **hydrocodone** PO.

Disposition   Release to home with follow-up in 3–5 days with an ear, nose, and throat specialist for further evaluation of hearing loss.

Epistaxis

Etiology
- Trauma, blood dyscrasia, hypertension

Nursing Diagnoses
- Risk for fluid volume deficit

Common Complaints
- Bloody nose

Triage Rating
- Urgent to emergent

Related Factors
- Epistaxis can occur in either the anterior or posterior area of the nasal passage. Anterior bleeding is most common and more frequent during the winter months. Posterior bleeding occurs more commonly in the elderly population. Epistaxis is rare in hemophiliacs without associated injury but is a characteristic of von Willebrand's disease. Intranasal foreign objects can also cause nasal bleeding.

Assessment Findings
- Fresh or dried blood in nostril(s)
- Fresh blood in oropharynx associated with posterior bleeding
- Blood pressure: may be normal, low, or elevated
- Tachycardia

Diagnostics
- CBC: possible lowered hemoglobin and hematocrit

Interventions
- Apply pressure over anterior nasal septum for 10–15 minutes.
- Position patient sitting up and leaning forward.
- Gently suction nose with nasal suction equipment.
- Apply topical medications to control bleeding:
  - **Epinephrine** 1:1000.
  - **Phenylephrine** 1%.
  - **Lidocaine** 4% *or* **cocaine** 4%.
- Assist with other treatments to control bleeding:
  - Electric cauterization of site.
  - Silver nitrate stick to site.
  - Anterior nasal pack with possible agent such as **Oxicel**, **Gelfoam**, **Surgicel**, **Avitene**, or **Merocel** nasal tampon.
  - Posterior nasal pack placed by ear, nose, and throat specialist.
- Consider insertion of IV and infuse NS fluids.
- Obtain blood samples for CBC, PT and PTT studies.
- Monitor continued blood loss, BP, pulse rate and rhythm, respiratory rate, pulse oximetry.

Disposition   Patients with anterior nasal bleeding that is controlled in the ED can be released to home. Instructions should include how to manage nasal bleeding at home, how to increase humidity in the home during winter months, and use of lubricant to the nares to prevent drying of the mucous membranes.

Patients with posterior nasal bleeding require hospital admission.

Nasal Foreign Object

Etiology
- Intentional insertion of object into nasal passage

Nursing Diagnoses
- Pain

Common Complaints
- Sneezing, unilateral nasal discharge

Triage Rating
- Nonurgent

Related Factors
- This condition usually occurs in children, especially in children <4 years of age. The most common underlying identifying factor is a history of chronic rhinitis.

Assessment Findings
- Occluded nasal passage with visible foreign object
- Unilateral rhinitis
- Possible foul odor from nares

Diagnostics
- None

Interventions
- Attempt removal using alligator forceps or gentle suction.
- If unsuccessful have parent occlude patient's unaffected nostril, then forcefully blow air into the child's mouth *or* if child is old enough to follow directions, have the child occlude the unaffected nostril, close lips, and forcefully blow air out the affected nostril.

Disposition   Release to home if object is removed. If the object cannot be removed in the ED, refer to ear, nose, and throat specialist for possible hospitalization and surgical removal.

Sinusitis

Etiology
- Bacterial, virus, or fungal organism

Nursing Diagnoses
- Pain
- Infection

Common Complaints
- Headache, fever, sinus pain that increases with forward bending or coughing

Triage Rating
- Nonurgent to emergent

Related Factors
- May be acute or chronic and involves inflammation of the paranasal sinuses. Sinusitis may follow a recent upper respiratory tract infection, dental abscess, or allergy. The most common causing bacterial organisms include *Streptococcus pneumoniae*, *Haemophilus influenzae*, and *Moraxella catarrhalis*. Maxillary sinusitus is the major site of infection in children.

Assessment Findings
- Possible periorbital swelling
- Tenderness over affected sinus
- Swollen, inflamed nasal mucosa
- Postnasal discharge

Diagnostics
- Radiographic studies: sinus films or Waters' projection may demonstrate air fluid levels, opacification of affected sinus, or thickening of sinus

Interventions
- Administer antibiotic medication:
  - **Amoxicillin** 125–500 mg PO *or* **amoxicillin-clavulanate** 125–250 mg PO.
  - **Cefuroxime** 500 mg–1.5 g (Peds: 75–150 mg/kg/d) IV if preseptal or periorbital cellulitis present.

Disposition   Release to home with follow-up in 24–48 hours. Instruct patient to increase fluids and use topical decongestants for 3–4 days. Consider hospitalization for aggressive antibiotic therapy if preseptal or periorbital cellulitis is present.

Ludwig's Angina

Etiology
- Bacterial organism

Nursing Diagnoses
- Pain
- Infection
- Risk for ineffective airway clearance

Common Complaints
- Pain in the jaw and neck, fever, difficulty swallowing

Triage Rating
- Urgent to emergent

Related Factors
- This infection is a septic cellulitis located around the submandibular gland, beneath the jaw and the floor of the mouth. The streptococcal bacilli is the common offending organism. The infection follows a descending pattern. It is an infection that more often affects elderly, debilitated men.

Assessment Findings
- Bilateral swelling of jaw and neck
- Elevated tongue
- Dyspnea and tachypnea
- Increased temperature
- Diaphoretic skin

Diagnostics
- CBC: elevated WBC caused by infection
- Radiographic studies: soft tissue of the neck to differentiate epiglottitis

Interventions
- Maintain airway patency and administer oxygen 6–15 L via face mask.
- Assist with possible surgical airway procedure.
- Insert IV and infuse NS fluid.
- Obtain blood samples for CBC.
- Assist with possible incision and drainage of abscess in infected area.
- Administer antibiotic medication:
  - **Penicillin G** 200,000 U/kg/d IV infusion.
- Monitor airway patency, BP, pulse rate and rhythm, pulse oximetry, temperature.

Disposition Consultation with ear, nose, and throat specialist and admission to critical care area.

Pharyngitis/Tonsillitis

Etiology
- Bacterial, viral, or fungal organism

Nursing Diagnoses
- Pain
- Infection

Common Complaints
- Sore throat, fever

Triage Rating
- Nonurgent to urgent

Related Factors
- Most common bacterial organisms include group A β-hemolytic *Streptococcus* and *Neisseria gonorrhoeae*. Other causes include coxsackievirus, echovirus, Epstein-Barr virus, and *Candida albicans*. Exudative pharyngitis can occur with either a virus or bacterial offending organism. Peritonsillar abscess is a complication of tonsillitis and requires aggressive treatment to minimize or prevent airway compromise.

Assessment Findings
- Increased temperature
- Posterior pharynx findings:
  - Erythema
  - Tonsil enlargement
  - Exudate with *Streptococcus* and Epstein-Barr virus
  - Ulcer lesions with coxsackievirus and echovirus
  - Palatal petechiae with Epstein-Barr virus
  - Swelling, bulging of tonsil in anterior pillar and possible uvular displacement with abcess
- Vesicle, ulcer lesions on hands and feet with coxsackievirus
- Tender cervical lymphadenopathy
- Drooling, muffled voice, trismus with abscess
- Other system assessments:
  - Heart tones for possible murmur
  - Abdomen for possible splenic enlargement
  - Skin for possible "sand paper" or petechiae rash
  - Neck for meningimus

Diagnostics
- Throat culture or rapid strep screen: positive with group A β-hemolytic *Streptococcus* if strep throat

Interventions
- Obtain throat culture if indicated.
- No antibiotic treatment for coxsackievirus, echovirus, or Epstein-Barr virus.
- Administer antibiotic medications for other pharyngitis:
  - **Penicillin** 250–500 mg PO *or* **benzathine LA** 600,000–1.2 million units IM.
  - **Erythromycin** 250–500 mg PO if allergic to penicillin.
  - **Ceftriaxone** 250 mg–1 g IM/IV infusion if suspected gonorrhea organism.
- Assist with possible incision and drainage if abscess is present.

Disposition   Release to home if stridor or drooling is not present with follow-up in 3–5 days. Instruct patient to increase fluid intake. Symptomatic pain relief may be obtained with throat lozenges, hard candies, and warm salt water gargles. Patients with difficulty swallowing secretions, drooling, or stridor must be hospitalized for monitoring of airway patency and aggressive therapy.

Stomatitis

Etiology
- Bacterial, viral, fungal organisms

Nursing Diagnoses
- Pain
- Infection

Common Complaints
- Oral pain or burning, sore throat, decreased food or fluid intake

Triage Rating
- Nonurgent to urgent

Related Factors
- Offending organisms include *Herpes simplex, Candida albicans,* coxsackie or echovirus, *Bacillus fusobacterium,* and *Borrelia vincentii.* This condition may be related to nutritional deficiencies (vitamin B_{12}, folate, or iron), tobacco, eating hot foods, systemic illness such as syphilis or leukemia, or localized allergic reactions. Primary herpetic stomatitis usually occurs in children 1–5 years of age, with secondary stomatitis more frequent in young adults to adult ages. Herpangina is common in children. Vincent's stomatitis is more frequent in teens and adults.

Assessment Findings
- Primary herpetic stomatitis:
  - Vesicles and ulcers with yellow-gray membrane on erythematous base located on pharynx, tonsils, soft palate
  - Anterior cervical adenopathy
  - Increased temperature
- Secondary herpetic stomatitis:
  - 24–48-hour prodrome of burning sensation
  - Vesicles and ulcers often at vermilion border of lips
  - Crusting may be present
- Herpangina:
  - Increased temperature
  - Papule, vesicle, ulcer lesions on anterior tonsil, pharynx, buccal mucosa
- Vincent's stomatitis:
  - Ulcers on gingivae and covered with purulent, gray exudate

Diagnostics
- Usually none

Interventions
- Administer pain relief medications:
  - **Lidocaine (Xylocaine)** viscous solution as mouthwash or apply to lesions *or* **diphenhydramine** elixir mixed with **lidocaine (Xylocaine)** viscous solution, **attapulgite**, **aluminum** or **magnesium hydroxide** applied to lesions.
- Consider administration of additional medications:
  - Herpetic stomatitis:
    - **Acyclovir** 400 mg PO.
  - Vincent's stomatitis:
    - **Penicillin** 250–500 mg PO.

Disposition
Release to home. Increase fluid intake, especially in children.

Asthma

Etiology
- Airway inflammation from external stimuli, bacterial or viral organisms, allergy

Nursing Diagnoses
- Ineffective breathing pattern
- Impaired gas exchange
- Ineffective airway clearance

Common Complaints
- Wheezing, cough, dyspnea, chest tightness

Triage Rating
- Urgent to emergent

Related Factors
- Stimuli that can produce inflammation, hyperresponsiveness, and narrowing of the airway are multiple. Aggravating factors include infection, medications, allergens, emotional upset, exercise, and environmental irritants. This disease is chronic with acute reversible exacerbations and affects 5–10% of children under the age of 20 years. The respiratory syncytial virus (RSV) is the most common cause in children <6 months of age. Persons >55years of age have the highest death rates from asthma.

Assessment Findings
- Restlessness
- Tachypnea
- Accessory muscle use
- Nasal flaring
- Wheezes: bilateral or unilateral*
- Tachycardia
- Pale, cool skin
- Pulse oximetry <94%
- Possible increased temperature

Diagnostics
- Peak flow reading before and after treatment: increase of 15–20% after treatment confirms diagnosis
- Radiographic studies: chest film may indicate hyperinflation, pneumonia, atelectasis
- ABG: PaO_2 low, $PaCO_2$ <35 mm Hg early in acute episode, >45 mm Hg later or in severe episode
- ECG: tachycardia; in adults possible right bundle branch block
- CBC: increased WBC if infection is present
- Theophylline level: normal, increased, or decreased

Interventions
- Position patient to facilitate breathing.
- Assist with intubation and mechanical ventilation if severe episode or status asthmaticus.
- Administer oxygen at 6–15 L via face mask.
- Administer bronchodilator medications:
  –**Albuterol** 0.25–0.5 mL in 2–3 mL of NS by nebulizer treatment *or* **metaproterenol** 0.1–0.3 mL in 2.5 mL NS intermittent (q20min) or continuous therapy.
  –**Epinephrine** 1:1000 0.3 mg (Peds: 0.01 mg/kg) SC.†
- Insert IV or saline lock.
- Obtain blood samples for CBC, serum medication levels, ABG.
- Administer additional medications if episode not responsive:
  –**Prednisolone** 5 mg/mL or 15 mg/mL PO *or* **prednisone** 60 mg PO.
  –**Methylprednisolone** 1–2 mg/kg IV.
  –**Aminophylline** 6 mg/kg loading dose IV infusion.
- Monitor respiratory rate, effort, and presence of wheezing, pulse oximetry, peak flow readings, BP, pulse rate and rhythm, level of consciousness.

*If wheezing is unilateral, consider inhalation of foreign object. Air trapping will be visible on chest film.
†Contraindicated in adults >35 years of age because of cardiac effects.

Disposition   If condition improves, release patient to home. If condition does not respond to therapy, hospitalization is necessary.

Bronchiolitis

Etiology
- Bacterial or viral organism

Nursing Diagnoses
- Ineffective breathing pattern
- Impaired gas exchange
- Risk for infection

Common Complaints
- Poor feeding, wheezing, rapid respiratory rate, fever

Triage Rating
- Urgent

Related Factors
- Causative organisms include respiratory syncytial virus (RSV), parainfluenza, adenovirus, enterovirus, and less frequently *Mycoplasma pneumoniae*. Usual age group is infant <24 months of age, with boys affected at a 2:1 ratio. Occurrences are usually in late winter or early spring.

Assessment Findings
- Respiratory distress with nasal flaring, intercostal or subcostal retractions, and use of accessory muscles
- Tachypnea
- Wheezes, crackles, or rhonchi
- Pulse oximetry <94%
- Tachycardia
- Vomiting
- Possible listlessness and cyanosis

Diagnostics
- Radiographic studies: chest film indicating hyperinflation, flattened or depressed diaphragm, scattered areas of atelectasis, perihilar infiltrates, and hilar adenopathy
- CBC: increased WBC if infection present
- Serum chemistries: possibly altered indicating dehydration
- Nasal washing for collection of RSV pathogen

Interventions
- Position patient with head elevated.
- Administer oxygen at flow rate to maintain pulse oximetry >95%. Deliver by mist tent, blow-by, nasal cannula, or face mask.
- Insert IV or saline lock. Use buritrol chamber and infuse D5.25 NS fluid.
- Obtain blood samples for CBC, chemistries.
- Obtain nasal washing.
- Administer bronchodilator medications:
  –**Albuterol** 0.1–0.15 mg/kg in 2 mL NS nebulizer for intermittent treatment q20min or continuous treatment.
- Monitor respiratory rate and effort, presence of wheezes or rhonchi, pulse oximetry, BP, pulse rate, fluid intake and output.

Disposition   With moderate to severe cases hospitalization is necessary. Children with mild cases of bronchiolitis may be released to home with follow-up within 24 hours.

Bronchitis

Etiology
- Bacterial or viral organism

Nursing Diagnoses
- Ineffective breathing pattern
- Impaired gas exchange
- Risk for infection

Common Complaints
- Cough, chest pain, wheezing, white sputum production, fever

Triage Rating
- Nonurgent to urgent

Related Factors
- Often results from primary infection of cold viruses, influenza, adenovirus, *Mycoplasma pneumoniae, Chlamydia pneumoniae,* or *Moraxella catarrhalis.* A history of smoking is frequently present. Bronchitis commonly occurs in young healthy males, but may also appear in the elderly population who have underlying pulmonary disease. Bronchitis is often a diagnosis of exclusion.

Assessment Findings
- Slight tachypnea
- Scattered rhonchi that clear with coughing
- Pulse oximetry: normal to slight decrease
- Possible increased temperature

Diagnostics
- Radiographic studies: chest film often is normal, or hyperinflation and perihilar infiltration may be present

Interventions
- Administer or prescribe antibiotic medication if patient smokes:
  - **Erythromycin** 250–500 mg PO.

Disposition　Release to home with follow-up in 3–5 days.

Chronic Obstructive Pulmonary Disease

Etiology
- Smoking or environmental agents that destroy lung parenchyma

Nursing Diagnoses
- Ineffective breathing pattern
- Impaired gas exchange

Common Complaints
- Fatigue, shortness of breath, chronic productive cough, fever

Triage Rating
- Urgent

Related Factors
- A chronic, nonreversible pulmonary disease that reduces the elastic recoil of the lungs. It is most frequently associated with a smoking history and often begins early in adult life. Over time, the patient's condition worsens. Infection can lead to acute respiratory failure and death.

Assessment Findings
- Restlessness
- Tachypnea
- Pale or cyanotic color
- Pursed lip breathing
- Accessory muscle use to breathe
- Inability to speak and breathe at the same time
- Diminished breath sounds with wheezes, rales, or rhonchi
- Hyperresonant percussion sounds in chest
- Pulse oximetry <94%
- Tachycardia
- Possible increased temperature

Diagnostics
- Radiographic studies: chest films may demonstrate flattened diaphragm, hyperinflation, right ventricular enlargement, and increased AP diameter; possible infectious process
- ECG: irregular rhythm with ectopy such as PVCs or bundle branch block
- CBC: elevated WBC if infection present
- Sputum culture: results unavailable for 24–48 hours
- ABG: if obtained O_2 <80 mm Hg, $Paco_2$ >45 mm Hg

Interventions
- Position patient to facilitate breathing.
- Administer oxygen 2–15 L via nasal cannula or face mask.
- Insert IV or saline lock.
- Obtain blood samples for CBC and other studies.
- Administer bronchodilator medications:
  –**Metaproterenol** 0.2–0.3 mL in 2–3 mL NS *or* **albuterol** 0.5 mL in 2–3 mL NS for nebulizer treatment continuous or intermittent (q20min).
  –Compressed air may be used to decrease the amount of inspired air.
- Administer antibiotic medication as needed:
  –**Erythromycin** 500 mg PO.
- Monitor level of consciousness, BP, pulse rate and rhythm, respiratory rate and effort, pulse oximetry.

Disposition   Release to home if respiratory rate and effort return to normal for the patient. If respiratory distress develops or is not relieved, hospitalization is required.

Croup (Laryngotracheobronchitis)

Etiology
• Viral organism or allergy

Nursing Diagnoses
• Risk for ineffective airway clearance

Common Complaints
• "Barky" cough or hoarseness usually occurring at night

Triage Rating
• Urgent to emergent

Related Factors
• Common in children of all ages and often occurs following an upper respiratory infection. The usual offending organisms are the parainfluenza, respiratory syncytial virus (RSV), or *Mycoplasma pneumoniae*. The episodes can range from mild to severe; however, symptoms usually abate within 3–7 days.

Assessment Findings
• Restlessness or irritability
• "Barky" cough or stridor
• Accessory muscle use or nasal flaring
• Intercostal retractions
• Tachypnea
• Clear but diminished breath sounds
• Temperature <103°F

Diagnostics
• Radiographic studies: soft tissue of the neck may demonstrate a steeple sign

Interventions
• Administer humidified oxygen 6–10 L flow rate, may be administered via blow-by.
• Administer steroid medication: –**Prednisolone** 5 mg/mL or 15 mg/mL PO.
• If not responsive, consider administration of: –**Racemic epinephrine***
0.25–0.50 of 2.25% solution in 3 mL NS via nebulizer.
• Monitor level of consciousness, respiratory rate and effort, pulse rate, BP.

*If administered, child requires observation or hospitalization because of the rebound effects of racemic epinephrine.

Disposition   The majority of children can be released to home. Instruct parents to humidify the air at home.

Epiglottitis

Etiology
- Bacterial organism

Nursing Diagnoses
- Risk for ineffective airway clearance

Common Complaints
- Fever, drooling, dysphagia, dysphonia

Triage Rating
- Emergent

Related Factors
- *Haemophilus influenzae* type B is the causative organism. The epiglottis and surrounding structures become inflamed and edematous, producing a rapidly progressing respiratory emergency. Although this can occur at any age, it is most common in boys ages 3–7 years.

Assessment Findings
- Ill-appearing child
- Increased temperature
- Drooling
- Inspiratory stridor
- Nasal flaring
- Child positioned in sitting forward or "sniffing" position, jaw thrust forward
- Pale or cyanotic color
- Tachycardia

Diagnostics
- Radiographic studies: soft tissue of the neck showing an enlarged epiglottis or "thumb sign"
- CBC: elevated WBC

Interventions
- Allow patient to remain in position that facilitates airway patency.
- Assist with intubation as needed to maintain airway patency and deliver humidified cool oxygen.
- Insert IV and infuse* D5.2 NS fluids.
- Obtain blood* samples for CBC and other studies.
- Administer antibiotic medication:*
  –**Cefuroxime** 75–150 mg/kg IV infusion *or* **cefotaxime** 100–200 mg/kg IV infusion *or* **chloramphenicol** 100–200 mg/kg IV infusion.

*Invasive procedures should be performed only after airway stabilization has occurred.

Disposition   Hospitalization to pediatric critical care area. If intubation is required and is not performed in the ED, admission to the operating room suite may be required for the intubation procedure.

Hyperventilation (Anxiety Related)

Etiology
- Anxiety

Nursing Diagnoses
- Ineffective breathing pattern
- Impaired gas exchange
- Anxiety

Common Complaints
- Chest pain, carpopedal spasms, tingling of lips, breathlessness if caused by anxiety

Triage Rating
- Nonurgent (urgent, emergent if nonanxiety related)

Related Factors
- An increase in respiratory rate and depth results in a decrease in $Paco_2$. The underlying cause for the alteration in respirations must be quickly determined. Anxiety is a common cause, but other causes such as increased ICP, acute MI, pulmonary emboli, or metabolic disorders must be considered before the beginning of treatment. If the cause is a condition other than anxiety, treatment to correct the underlying problem is the priority.

Assessment Findings
- Tachypnea
- Pale skin
- Spasms of the hands and feet
- Tachycardia

Diagnostics
- Usually none

Interventions
- Instruct patient to take slow deep breaths through the nose and exhale through the mouth.
- Consider having patient breathe into a paper bag.
- Monitor respiratory rate and depth, relief of chest pain and carpopedal spasms, skin color, pulse rate, BP.

Disposition   Release to home when symptoms have abated. Instruct the patient in rebreathing techniques should future episodes occur.

Pleurisy

Etiology
- Trauma, viral or bacterial organism

Nursing Diagnoses
- Pain
- Ineffective breathing pattern

Common Complaints
- Chest pain made worse by inspiration or sudden thoracic movements

Triage Rating
- Nonurgent

Related Factors
- Bronchitis is a common cause of pleurisy. This condition occurs when the pleural surface becomes inflamed. The onset may be gradual or sudden.

Assessment Findings
- Tachypnea with shallow depth
- Respiratory splinting
- Pleural friction rub
- Possible rales, rhonchi, or wheezing

Diagnostics
- CBC: WBC elevated with infection
- Radiographic studies: chest film shows no acute pathology
- V/Q scan: normal if symptoms not caused by pulmonary emboli

Interventions
- Administer pain medication:
  –**Acetaminophen with codeine** *or* **hydrocodone** PO.
- Administer antiinflammatory medications:
  –**NSAIDs** (e.g., **ibuprofen** 600–800 mg) PO.

Disposition Release to home.

Pneumonia

Etiology
- Bacterial, viral, fungal organism; aspiration

Nursing Diagnoses
- Infection
- Impaired gas exchange

Common Complaints
- Cough, fever, sputum production

Triage Rating
- Nonurgent to urgent

Related Factors
- Infection of the lung parenchyma, interstitial tissue, and alveolar spaces. Common age-related organisms: <3 months of age—*Chlamydia trachomatis*, respiratory syncytial virus (RSV), or genital mycoplasmas; 3 months–5 years of age—RSV, *Streptococcus pneumoniae* or *Haemophilus influenzae* type B; older children—*Mycoplasma pneumoniae, Streptococcus pneumoniae, Chlamydia pneumoniae,* or viruses; Adults—any of these bacteria or viruses, in addition to *Staphylococcus, Legionella pneumophila,* or *Mycobacterium tuberculosis.* Immunocompromised patients frequently develop pneumonia from cytomegalovirus or *Pneumocystis carinii.* In adults pneumonia is the sixth leading cause of death. Pneumonia with fever during pregnancy may lead to premature labor. Varicella pneumonia during pregnancy carries a 45% mortality rate.

Assessment Findings
- Possible restlessness
- Increased temperature
- Tachypnea
- Dull areas in the chest with percussion
- Bronchial or rhonchi lung sounds with localized diminished sounds
- Tachycardia
- Sputum production with cough
- Pulse oximetry may be <94%

Diagnostics
- Radiographic studies: chest film findings will vary depending on causative organisms*
- Sputum gram stain and culture: helpful with *Mycobacterium, Legionella,* and endemic fungi
- CBC:[†] WBC elevated if bacterial pneumonia
- Other blood tests:[†] electrolytes, hepatic enzymes, renal function, blood culture
- Consider tuberculosis skin test

Interventions
- Administer oxygen at flow rate to maintain pulse oximetry >95%.
- Position patient to facilitate breathing.
- Insert IV and infuse NS fluids.
- Obtain blood samples for CBC, chemistries, and other tests.
- Administer antibiotic medication depending on suspected causative organism.[‡]
- Monitor respiratory rate and effort, pulse rate and rhythm, pulse oximetry, BP, urinary output, restlessness.

*Chest film findings:
- Lobar or segmental infiltrates with *Streptococcus pneumoniae, Haemophilus influenzae, Klebsiella, Escherichia coli, Legionella*
- Patchy or streaky opacities with *Mycoplasma pneumoniae,* viruses, *Legionella*
- Diffuse homogenous infiltrates with *Legionella,* viruses, *Pneumocystis carinii* pneumonia
- Nodular opacities with *Mycobacterium, Aspergillus, Candida*
- Cavity infiltrates with *Staphylococcus aureus, Mycobacterium tuberculosis, Aspergillus*

[†]Consider laboratory tests in patients >60 years of age.

[‡]Antibiotic therapy depending on causative organism:
- *Pneumococcal* pneumonia: **Penicillin V** 250–500 mg qid 7–10 days or 300,000 units IM as first dose. Alternative: **erythromycin** 250–500 mg qid 7–10 days, or **azithromycin** 500 mg on the first day then 250 mg qd for 4 days
- *Haemophilus influenzae, Moraxella catarrhalis,* staphylococcus, gram-negative bacilli: **Amoxicillin-clavulanate** 250–500 mg tid 10 days, **cefuroxime** 250–500 mg bid 10 days, or **ciprofloxacin** 200 mg bid 10 days
- *Mycoplasma pneumoniae, Chlamydia pneumoniae*: **Doxycycline** 100 mg bid for 10–14 days, or **erythromycin** 250–500 mg tid 10–14 days
- *Legionella*: **Erythromycin** 1 g IV qid, **doxycycline** 100 mg qd 14 days, or **ciprofloxacin** 200 mg bid 10–14 days
- *Pneumocystis carinii*: **Trimethoprim-sulfamethoxazole** 20 mg/kg/d IV qid doses, or 100 mg/kg/d in qid dose 14–21 days

Disposition
Release to home if mild symptoms. Patients moderately to severely ill require hospitalization; consider hospitalization in infants <2 months, adults >60 years of age, or persons with coexisting illness.

Pneumothorax (Simple or Spontaneous)

Etiology
- Trauma, cough

Nursing Diagnoses
- Pain
- Ineffective breathing pattern

Common Complaints
- Sudden sharp chest pain, shortness of breath, pain to the ipsilateral shoulder

Triage Rating
- Urgent

Related Factors
- A history of smoking is common with the development of a spontaneous or primary pneumothorax. This occurs more frequently in thin men, beginning in the third decade of life. Barotrauma, underlying pulmonary disease, or a sudden increase in intrathoracic pressure may also be the precipitating cause.

Assessment Findings
- Restlessness
- Tachypnea with shallow respiratory effort
- Diminished breath sounds over area of pneumothorax
- Hyperresonant percussion sounds over area of pneumothorax
- Pulse oximetry <94% to normal

Diagnostics
- Radiographic studies: chest film indicating presence of pneumothorax (thin visceral pleural line displaced away from chest wall)

Interventions
- Administer oxygen 2–6 L via nasal cannula.
- If pneumothorax is >10% assist with chest tube insertion and attach to chest drainage container.
- Monitor respiratory rate and effort, pulse rate and rhythm, BP, level of consciousness.

Disposition   Admission to hospital is required if the pneumothorax size required the insertion of a chest tube for reexpansion. If a chest tube is not required, release to home with follow-up within 24 hours for a second chest film.

Pulmonary Edema (Congestive Heart Failure)

Etiology
- Cardiac failure, inhalation injury, near drowning, sepsis, narcotic overdose, trauma

Nursing Diagnoses
- Ineffective breathing pattern
- Impaired gas exchange
- Fluid volume overload

Common Complaints
- Difficulty breathing, chest pain, diaphoresis

Triage Rating
- Emergent

Related Factors
- With cardiac related pulmonary edema, the left ventricle has been damaged. Ejection fraction decreases, and pressure in the left ventricle increases. Over time, this pressure increase eventually affects the left atria and right ventricle and atria. Pulmonary edema occurring from noncardiac origins is the result of acute damage to the alveolocapillary membrane. As permeability increases, fluid collects in the interstitial space, surfactant levels decrease, and eventually alveoli collapse.

Assessment Findings
- Restlessness, decreased level of consciousness
- Tachypnea with increased respiratory effort
- Respiratory rales
- Pale, cyanotic, diaphoretic skin
- Distended jugular veins
- Tachycardia
- Hypertension or hypotension
- Pulse oximetry <94%
- Pitting-dependent edema, ascites

Diagnostics
- ABG: pH >7.45 (alkalosis), Pao_2 <80 mm Hg, $Paco_2$ <35 mm Hg (respiratory alkalosis)
- Laboratory studies: CBC, chemistries, digitalis level
- Radiographic studies: chest film demonstrates interstitial infiltrates; also will confirm intubation tube placement
- ECG: tachycardia with possible dysrhythmia

Interventions
- Position patient upright to facilitate breathing.
- Administer oxygen 6–15 L via face mask.
- Intubation if respiratory fatigue or failure develops with mechanical ventilation.
- Insert IV or saline lock.
- Obtain blood samples for CBC, chemistries, and other studies.
- Insert nasogastric tube and attach to suction.
- Insert indwelling urinary catheter.
- Administer medications to decrease fluid overload:
  –**Nitroglycerin** 5–10 µg/min IV infusion and titrated to patient response.
  –**Furosemide** 20–100 mg IV.
  –**Morphine sulfate** 2–10 mg IV.
- Administer medications to augment cardiac output:
  –**Digoxin*** 0.6–1 mg IV.
- Monitor level of consciousness, respiratory rate and effort, pulse oximetry, pulse rate and rhythm, BP, intake and urinary output.

*Before administering digoxin, serum digoxin and potassium levels must be known to prevent digoxin toxicity.

Disposition   Majority of patients require hospital admission for continued monitoring and therapy. Only those patients with mild pulmonary edema should be considered for outpatient management.

Pulmonary Emboli

Etiology
- Recent trauma, childbirth, deep water diving, cardiac atrial fibrillation, deep vein thrombosis

Nursing Diagnoses
- Altered tissue perfusion: pulmonary
- Ineffective breathing pattern
- Impaired gas exchange

Common Complaints
- Shortness of breath, chest pain, cough

Triage Rating
- Urgent to emergent

Related Factors
- Occlusion of the pulmonary arterial circulation results in the shunting of blood flow and an alteration in the pulmonary V/Q ratio. Occlusion occurs from foreign material or a thromboembolus that traveled from a systemic vein. Emboli may develop from air, amniotic fluid, or blood clots. Risk factors associated with the development of an emboli include prolonged immobilization, thrombophlebitis, recent surgery, recent childbirth, use of birth control pills, obesity, recent MI, atrial fibrillation, or congestive heart failure.

Assessment Findings
- Restlessness
- Tachypnea
- Pulse oximetry <94%
- Breath sounds: clear or crackles, wheezing may be present
- Tachycardia
- Possible swelling of lower extremity

Diagnostics
- Radiographic studies: chest film usually normal, or elevated diaphragm may be noted; V/Q scan indicating multiple segment mismatch; Doppler ultrasound or lower extremity venogram may indicate deep vein thrombosis
- ECG: tachycardia; elevated ST segment; large P wave in leads II, III, aVF; inverted T waves in leads V_1, V_4
- Laboratory studies: CBC, PT, PTT for baseline
- ABG: pH >7.45 (alkalosis), Pao_2 decreased, $Paco_2$ <35 mm Hg (respiratory alkalosis)

Interventions
- Administer oxygen at flow rate to maintain pulse oximetry >94%.
- Insert IV or saline lock.
- Obtain blood samples for CBC, PT, PTT, and other studies.
- Administer thrombolytic medications:
  –**Heparin** 5000–10,000 units IV then 1000 U/h IV infusion.
  –**Alteplase** 100 mg IV over 2 hours divided bolus or continuous infusion *or* **streptokinase** 250,000 units IV over 30 minutes then 100,000 U/h.
- Monitor level of consciousness, pulse oximetry, respiratory rate and effort, breath sounds, pulse rate and rhythm, BP, development of oozing of blood.

Disposition   Admission to critical care area.

Simple Rib Fracture

Etiology
- Trauma

Nursing Diagnoses
- Pain
- Ineffective breathing pattern

Common Complaints
- Chest pain that increases with respirations

Triage Rating
- Nonurgent

Related Factors
- A common type of chest injury usually from blunt forces. A fracture of ribs 1 or 2 is associated with significant injury in addition to concomitant fractures of the clavicle and scapula. Rib fracture of the lower left or right thoracic cage may be associated with liver or splenic injuries. The majority of rib fractures are of minor consequence. Children are less likely to sustain rib fractures from blunt forces to the chest because of the flexibility of the rib cage.

Assessment Findings
- Hypoventilation caused by pain
- Tenderness over injury site
- Possible palpable crepitus over fracture site

Diagnostics
- Radiographic studies: chest film may not identify area of fracture, of concern is presence of pneumothorax

Interventions
- Administer medication to relieve pain:
  - **Acetaminophen with codeine** *or* **hydrocodone** PO.
- Assist with possible intercostal nerve block.

Disposition   Release to home unless other injuries are present. Instruct patient to cough and deep breathe 1 or 2 times each hour. Do not provide patient with restrictive belts or binders that inhibit respiratory excursion.

Tietze's Syndrome (Costal Chondritis)

Etiology
- Trauma or overuse

Nursing Diagnoses
- Pain

Common Complaints
- Sharp, anterior chest pain

Triage Rating
- Nonurgent

Related Factors
- Usual areas affected are the costochondral or chondrosternal junction. Minor injury, heavy lifting, strenuous exercise, or severe coughing may be the precipitating factor. Pain is localized to the area of injury.

Assessment Findings
- Point tenderness over affected area
- Slight swelling over affected area
- Possible erythema of area

Diagnostics
- Radiographic studies: chest film usually demonstates no abnormalities

Interventions
- Administer antiinflammatory medications:
  –**Ibuprofen** 600–800 mg *or* other **NSAIDs** PO.

Disposition   Release to home.

Tuberculosis (Active)

Etiology
- *Mycobacterium tuberculosis* organism

Nursing Diagnoses
- Impaired gas exchange

Common Complaints
- Fatigue, weight loss, chronic cough, night sweats, fever, chest pain

Triage Rating
- Urgent

Related Factors
- The organism is spread through droplet nuclei from the respiratory tract. Between 90–95% of primary tuberculosis (TB) infections remain in the dormant stage and become active during times of stress, onset of diabetes, corticosteroid therapy, or in an immunocompromised host. The apical area of the lungs is the most common site for TB. The disease can lead to pleural effusions. Disseminated TB or infections of the lymphatic, genitourinary, skeletal, pericardial, or meningeal systems may also occur. Any adult person with TB should also be tested for HIV.

Assessment Findings
- Restlessness
- Possible thin, wasted appearance
- Increased temperature
- Tachypnea
- Rales in apical posterior lungs
- Blood-streaked sputum
- Pulse oximetry <94%
- Possible pericardial friction rub
- Tachycardia
- Possible enlarged cervical lymphadenopathy

Diagnostics
- Radiographic studies: chest film may demonstrate apical infiltrates, cavitary lesions, mediastinal or hilar adenopathy, atelectasis, pericardial calcification, or pleural effusions
- Sputum culture: results may require 3–6 weeks; acid-fast smear provides immediate positive/negative results
- Other cultures: from suspected sites
- Serum chemistry: may indicate calcium >5.3 mEq/L (total), sodium <135 mEq/L, hypoalbuminemia, abnormal liver function tests
- PPD test: positive*

Interventions
- Isolate patient from other ED patients.
- Place respiratory mask over patient, health care worker also must wear a mask that is fabricated to filter out droplet nuclei.
- Administer oxygen at flow rate to maintain pulse oximetry >94%.
- Insert IV and infuse NS fluid.
- Obtain blood samples for CBC, chemistries, and other studies.
- Administer antituberculin medications:
  –**Isoniazid**† 5 mg/kg (300 mg/d maximum) IM or PO (Peds: 10–20 mg/kg; 300 mg/d maximum).
  –Combined therapy including:
  - **Rifampin** 600 mg IV or PO.
  - **Pyrazinamide** 15–30 mg/kg (2 g maximum) PO.
  - **Ethambutol** 15–25 mg/kg (2.5 g maximum) PO.
- Monitor respiratory rate and effort, pulse oximetry, pulse rate and rhythm, BP, compliance with respiratory isolation.

*Positive PPD:
- >5 mm if patient HIV positive; has abnormal chest film; has had contact with another person with TB; is a child with positive symptoms of TB
- >10 mm if patient is foreign born; from TB endemic country; resides in medically poor area or long-term care facility; IV drug user; had medical risk factor such as diabetes, chronic obstructive pulmonary disease, alcoholism, end-stage renal disease, malnutrition, malignancy; child <4 years of age; health care worker
- >15 mm for all other patients

†Administer 25 mg of **pyridoxine** to prevent peripheral neuropathy.

Disposition   Admission to hospital required for patients with active TB and respiratory distress.

Acute Myocardial Infarction*

Etiology
- Trauma, coronary artery disease with arterial occlusion

Nursing Diagnoses
- Decreased cardiac output
- Altered tissue perfusion: cardiac
- Pain

Common Complaints
- Chest pain (dull, squeezing) occurring at rest, nausea, sweating, shortness of breath

Triage Rating
- Emergent

Related Factors
- Usually occurs in persons >40 years but can develop in younger ages. A history of coronary artery disease or previous infarction is frequently present. Other risk factors include hypertension, smoking, diabetes, family history, sedentary lifestyle, obesity, and hyperlipidemia. Cocaine use may also precipitate an infarction.

Assessment Findings
- Restlessness
- Pale, diaphoretic, skin
- Possible S_3, S_4 heart sounds
- Tachycardia
- Cardiac dysrhythmias: PVCs, bradycardia
- Pulmonary rales

Diagnostics
- ECG: abnormal Q waves, ST segment changes (elevation with acute MI, depression with ischemia), T wave changes, dysrhythmia
- Radiographic studies: chest film may show pulmonary congestion
- Cardic enzymes: elevated CK with elevation of isoenzyme CK-MB
- Myoglobin: may be elevated

Interventions
- Administer oxygen 6–15 L via face mask.
- Insert IV or saline locks: minimum of two lines.
- Obtain blood samples for CBC, chemistries, enzymes, PT, PTT, fibrinogen.
- Administer medications to improve cardiac output, muscle perfusion, decrease thrombi formation and pain:
  –**Aspirin** 80–85 mg chewable and enteric coated.
  –**Lidocaine** 1 mg/kg IV for PVCs, followed by 2 mg/min IV infusion.
  –Thrombolytic medication if patient meets criteria:[†]
  - **Streptokinase** 1.5 million units in 250 D5W IV infusion over 20 minutes *or* **alteplase** 15 mg IV followed by 50 mg IV infusion over 30 minutes, 35 mg over 1 hour *or* **anistreplase** 30 mg IV over 2 minutes.
  - **Heparin** 5000 units IV followed by 100 U/h IV infusion.
  - **Nitroglycerin** 0.4 mg SL q5min for 15 minutes or IV infusion of 50 mg in 250 mL DSW dilution and titrated at 5–10 µg/min to patient pain relief.
  - **Morphine sulfate** 2–4 mg IV and titrate to pain relief.
- Consider administration of β-blocker medication:
  –**Metoprolol** 5 mg IV over 2 minutes × 3 doses.
- Monitor level of consciousness, BP, pulse rate and rhythm, pulse oximetry, respiratory rate, pain relief.

*Other causes of chest pain include:
- Angina
- Pulmonary emboli
- Pneumothroax
- Pneumonia
- Esophagitis
- Pancreatitis
- Cholecystitis
- Chest musculoskeletal pain
- Pericarditis
- Mitral valve prolapse
- Aortic stenosis/insufficiency
- Aortic dissection
- Pleurisy

†Guidelines for administering thrombolytic therapy:
- Chest pain present for <6 hours
- <75 years of age
- No recent surgery, trauma, or cerebral vascular accident

Disposition
Admit for cardiac catheterization or to critical care area or if required transfer to regional cardiac center.

Angina

Etiology
- Coronary artery disease, coronary artery spasm

Nursing Diagnoses
- Pain
- Altered tissue perfusion: cardiac
- Decreased cardiac output

Common Complaints
- Chest pain or pressure that may radiate into the jaw, neck, or down the arms; usually lasts 2–10 minutes but not longer than 30 minutes

Triage Rating
- Urgent

Related Factors
- Angina pectoris is categorized as stable, unstable, or atypical. Angina occurs when the cardiac oxygen demand exceeds the oxygen supply. This may develop following exercise or an increased work load (stable angina) or at rest (unstable). These two types of angina are the result of coronary artery disease. Atypical or variant angina is associated with coronary artery spasm, and symptoms usually occur in a cyclic pattern. The pain identified with angina may also be similar to pain of other entities such as pulmonary embolism, aortic dissection, pericarditis, esophageal spasm, chest wall pain.

Assessment Findings
- Restlessness because of pain
- Hypertension
- Tachycardia
- Tachypnea, dyspnea
- Diaphoresis

Diagnostics
- ECG: T wave elevation without evidence of infarction; ST elevation may be present in variant angina during the time of pain
- Cardiac enzymes: normal

Interventions
- Administer oxygen 6–15 L via face mask or 2–6 L via nasal cannula.
- Insert IV or saline lock.
- Obtain blood samples for CBC, chemistries, cardiac enzymes, and other studies.
- Administer medications to restore tissue perfusion and relieve pain:
  –**Nitroglycerin** 0.4 mg SL repeated q5min for 15 minutes, or IV infusion of 50 mg in 250 mL D5W dilution and titrated at 5–10 µg/min to patient pain relief and maintaining the systolic BP >100 mm Hg.
  –Variant angina medications:
  - **Verapamil** 5–10 mg IV *or* **diltiazem** 0.25 mg/kg IV over 2 minutes or 5–15 mg/h IV infusion *or* **nifedipine** 10–40 mg PO/SL.
- Monitor level of consciousness, BP, pulse rate and rhythm, pulse oximetry, respiratory rate, and pain relief.

Disposition   If complete pain relief is achieved with treatment and angina is determined to be stable, patient may be released to home. Otherwise admission to telemetry or critical care area.

Aortic Aneurysm Dissection

Etiology
- Destruction of elastic fibers in vessel wall

Nursing Diagnoses
- Pain
- Risk for fluid volume deficit
- Altered tissue perfusion
- Decreased cardiac output

Common Complaints
- Chest, abdominal, back, or hip pain: may be unrelenting or described as sharp or tearing

Triage Rating
- Urgent to emergent

Related Factors
- Aneurysms may be classified as true, false, or dissecting. The most common site for aortic aneurysm is in the abdominal aorta below the renal arteries. True aneurysms are more common in men >60 years. Chronic hypertension is frequently present, but aneurysm may also be associated with Marfan syndrome, pregnancy, atherosclerosis, or trauma. If dissection or rupture occurs, hypovolemic shock will ensue.

Assessment Findings
- Restlessness, or decrease in level of consciousness
- Hypertension or hypotension
- Unequal blood pressure in upper arms
- Unequal pulses in extremities
- Tachycardia
- Tachypnea
- Diaphoresis
- Hemiplegia or paraplegia
- Possible heart murmur
- Peripheral cyanosis

Diagnostics
- Radiographic studies: chest film possibly demonstrating widening of the mediastinal shadow, abnormal aortic knob, aortic calcification, or a deviated trachea; aortogram indicating origin of the aneurysm or dissection; CT scan identifying the size and position of the aneurysm
- ECG: may show left ventricular hypertrophy; echocardiogram possibly identifying the size, shape, and location of the aneurysm
- CBC: usually not helpful unless rupture has occurred, then hemoglobin and hematocrit will be decreased
- Type and crossmatch for possible blood administration

Interventions
- Administer oxygen 6–15 L via face mask.
- Insert IV and infuse NS fluid. Consider infusion of colloid or blood.
- Obtain blood samples for CBC, chemistries, type and crossmatch, PT and PTT studies.
- Insert nasogastric tube and attach to suction.
- Insert indwelling urinary catheter.
- Administer medication to reduce blood pressure to between 100 and 200 mg Hg systolic: –**Nitroprusside** 0.25–8 µg/kg/min IV infusion *or* **labetalol** 2 mg/min or 20–40 mg q10–15min IV *or* **trimethaphan** 0.5–5 mg/min IV infusion.
- Administer medications to decrease force of myocardial contraction: –**Esmolol** loading dose 500 µg/kg/min followed by 25 µg/kg/min IV infusion *or* **propranolol** 0.5 mg IV followed by 1–2 mg q3–5min IV until pulse rate is between 60–75 bpm.
- Monitor level of consciousness, BP, pulse rate and rhythm, pulse oximetry, respiratory rate, urinary output.

Disposition   Admission to critical care area or to operating suite for possible surgical intervention.

Endocarditis

Etiology
- Bacterial, rickettsial, chlamydia, or fungal infection of the heart valves or endocardial heart surface

Nursing Diagnoses
- Infection
- Decreased cardiac output

Common Complaints
- Spiking fevers, malaise, night sweats, weight loss, arthralgias, and myalgias

Triage Rating
- Urgent

Related Factors
- Classified as either acute bacterial endocarditis (ABE) or subacute bacterial endocarditis (SBE). At-risk populations include IV drug users, patients with prosthetic heart valves or recent cardiac surgery, patients with congenital or rheumatic heart disease who have recently undergone invasive procedures without adequate antibiotic prophylaxis.* Congestive heart failure is a common complication.

Assessment Findings
- Temperature >102°F but may only be >99°F in SBE
- Heart murmur that increases with inspiration
- Tachycardia
- Fundoscopic examination: possible flame-shaped hemorrhages
- Warm, tender joint
- Petechiae on oropharynx and lower extremities
- Subungual splinter hemorrhage in the middle of the nail bed
- Osler's nodes: tender nodules on finger tips
- Janeway lesions: nonpainful patches on soles of the feet
- Splenomegaly

Diagnostics
- CBC: WBC may be normal with SBE but elevated with ABE
- Sedimentation rate: elevated
- Blood culture: positive in most cases
- Urinalysis: increased protein and microscopic hematuria
- ECG: possible conduction disturbance
- Radiographic studies: chest film possibly demonstrating pneumonia or pericardial effusion; echocardiography possibly indicating vegetative growth on valve leaflets

Interventions
- Administer oxygen 2–6 L via nasal cannula.
- Insert IV and infuse NS fluid.
- Obtain blood samples for CBC, blood cultures, sedimentation rate.
- Administer antibiotic medication: –**Penicillin G** 2 million units IV infusion *and* **streptomycin** 10 mg/kg (maximum 500 mg) IM *or* **gentamicin** 1.5 mg/kg IV infusion.
- Administer antipyretic medication: –**Acetaminophen** 650 mg PO.
- Monitor temperature, BP, pulse rate and rhythm.

*Suggested prophylactic antibiotic regimen for adult patients undergoing invasive surgery, instrumentation, or dental procedures:
- **Ampicillin** 2 g IM or IV + **gentamicin** 1.5 mg/kg (not to exceed 80 mg) IM or IV 30 minutes before procedure
- Penicillin-allergic patients:
  Vancomycin 1 g IV over 1 hour starting 1 hour before procedure + **gentamicin** 1.5 mg/kg (not to exceed 80 mg) IM 1 hour before procedure
- Low-risk procedures:
  Amoxicillin 3 g PO 1 hour before procedure

Disposition   Hospital admission to a critical care, telemetry, or medical unit.

Malignant Hypertension or Hypertensive Crisis

Etiology
- Chronic and progressive hypertension, pregnancy, Parnate-cheese reaction

Nursing Diagnoses
- Altered tissue perfusion
- Risk for injury

Common Complaints
- Severe headache associated with vomiting, visual changes, chest pain

Triage Rating
- Urgent to emergent

Related Factors
- Hypertension itself is not a disease but a physical finding indicating an underlying disease. As catecholamine levels increase, peripheral vasoconstriction occurs, elevating the BP. No specific BP measurement denotes hypertension, but diastolic pressure >130 mm Hg is associated with malignant hypertension. Adrenal tumor, sudden cessation of antihypertensive medication, pregnancy-induced hypertension (PIH), trauma, burns, and ingestion of tyramine in individuals taking MAO inhibitor medications are associated with malignant hypertension or crisis. Aggressively reducing the mean arterial pressure (MAP) below 90 mm Hg should be avoided as this can cause cerebral ischemia, especially in individuals with long-standing hypertension.

Assessment Findings
- Restlessness or decreased level of consciousness
- Possible seizure activity
- Elevated diastolic BP
- Fundoscopic examination: possible papilledema, hard exudates, linear hemorrhages

Diagnostics
- ECG: may indicate left ventricular strain and hypertrophy
- Radiographic studies: chest film possibly demonstrating enlarged heart and failure

Interventions
- Administer oxygen 2–6 L via nasal cannula.
- Insert IV or saline lock.
- Obtain blood samples for CBC, chemistries, and other studies.
- Administer antihypertensive medications:
  –**Nitroprusside** 0.25–8 µg/kg/min IV infusion.
  –**Labetalol** 2 mg/min IV infusion or 20 mg initially IV then 20–80 mg q10min.
  –**Hydralazine** (useful with PIH) 10–20 mg IV.
  –**Propranolol** 1–10 mg IV then 3 mg/h.
  –**Nifedipine** 10–20 mg PO or SL.
- Administer antiseizure medication if eclampsia (seizure activity) occurs with PIH:
  –**Magnesium sulfate** 1–4 g of 10–20% solution IV over 2–4 minutes or 5 g IV infusion at 1 g/h.
- Monitor level of consciousness, seizure activity, BP, pulse rate and rhythm, respiratory rate, pulse oximetry, motor movements, deep tendon reflexes, pain relief, urine output.

Disposition   Admission to critical care area or labor/delivery unit (for PIH) is required for patients with hypertensive emergencies. Patients with hypertensive urgent conditions may be admitted to a medical unit or may be released to home with close follow-up.

Malignant Hypertension or Hypertensive Crisis

Pericarditis

Etiology
- Viral, bacterial, fungal, chlamydia, rickettsial, or tuberculosis organisms

Nursing Diagnoses
- Infection
- Decreased cardiac output

Common Complaints
- Sharp, pleuritic chest pain that increases with respirations, may be referred to the neck or shoulder, and may decrease when patient leans forward; malaise; recent upper respiratory infection or gastrointestinal illness; fever; dyspnea

Triage Rating
- Urgent

Related Factors
- This inflammation of the pericardium or pericardial sac can be of an acute or chronic nature. It may also occur following an acute MI. Pericardial effusion and tamponade are other complications. Pericarditis can occur in children and is frequently caused by viral agents or rheumatic fever.

Assessment Findings
- Increased temperature
- Pericardial friction rub at Erb's point, which may increase in intensity when the patient leans forward
- Tachycardia
- Neck vein distension if effusion has developed

Diagnostics
- ECG: widespread ST elevation with corresponding ST depression in reciprocal leads; electrical alternans may be present with a large effusion
- Radiographic studies: chest film may demonstrate an enlarged cardiac silhouette if an effusion is present; echocardiogram demonstrating effusion if present

Interventions
- Administer oxygen 2–6 L via nasal cannula.
- Position patient in an upright, comfortable position.
- Administer antiinflammatory medications:
  –**Indomethacin** 25–50 mg PO.
  –**Ibuprofen** 400–800 mg PO.
- Assist with pericardiocentesis if large effusion present.
- Monitor pain relief, BP, pulse rate and rhythm, respiratory rate, pulse oximetry.

Disposition   Admission to hospital if effusion present or if pericardiocentesis was performed. Otherwise release to home.

Sinus Tachycardia

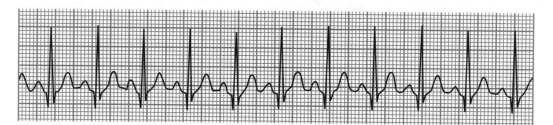

Characteristics

- Rate: >100 bpm
- Ventricular rhythm: regular
- P waves: present and uniformly shaped
- PR interval: between 0.12 and 0.2 seconds
- P wave/QRS relationship: P wave associated with each QRS complex
- QRS complex shape and width: uniformly shaped and between 0.08 and 0.1 seconds in duration
- Extra or abnormal beats: none

Treatment

- Eliminate the underlying cause.

Sinus Bradycardia

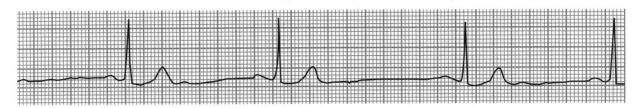

Characteristics

- Rate: <60 bpm
- Ventricular rhythm: regular
- P waves: present and uniformly shaped
- PR interval: usually between 0.12 and 0.2 seconds but may be prolonged
- P wave/QRS relationship: P wave associated with each QRS complex
- QRS complex shape and width: uniformly shaped and between 0.08 and 0.1 seconds in duration
- Extra or abnormal beats: usually none, but ventricular escape beats may occur

Treatment

- None if cardiac output is adequate.
- If hypotension, decreased level of consciousness, pale and diaphoretic skin, or chest pain are present, treatment is required:
  –Administer 100% oxygen.
  –Obtain venous access.
  –Administer **atropine** 0.5–1 mg IV and repeat q3–5min up to a maximum dose of 0.04 mg/kg.
  –Apply transcutaneous (external) cardiac pacing.
  –Administer **dopamine** 5–10 µg/kg/min IV infusion.
  –Administer **epinephrine** 2–10 µg/min IV infusion.
  –Administer **isoproterenol** IV infusion at low dose.
  –Consider transvenous cardiac pacing.

Paroxysmal Atrial Tachycardia (PAT)

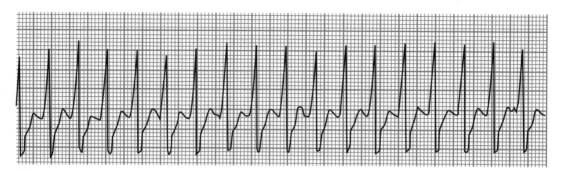

Characteristics

- Rate: >160 bpm
- Ventricular rhythm: regular
- P waves: present and uniformly shaped but may be hidden in the preceding T wave
- PR interval: between 0.12 and 0.2 seconds but may be difficult to determine
- P wave/QRS relationship: P wave associated with each QRS complex, but P wave may be difficult to identify
- QRS complex shape and width: uniformly shaped and between 0.08 and 0.1 seconds in duration
- Extra or abnormal beats: none

Treatment

- If rhythm does not spontaneously revert to regular sinus rhythm, treatment is required:
  –Administer oxygen.
  –Begin vagal stimulation (Valsalva's maneuver/carotid sinus massage).
  –Obtain venous access.
  –Administer **adenosine** 6–12 mg rapid IV, followed immediately with 20–30 mL fluid flush. May repeat × 1.
- If rhythm is not converted consider administering:
  –**Verapamil** 5–10 mg IV over 2 minutes.
  –**Lidocaine** 1–1.5 mg/kg up to a maximum of 3 mg/kg or **procainamide** 20–30 mg/min up to a maximum of 17 mg/kg.
  –**Magnesium sulfate** 1–2 g IV.
  –Medication failure to convert rhythm necessitates further treatment with synchronized cardioversion.

Atrial Flutter

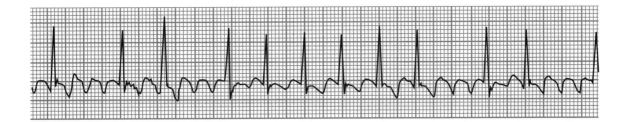

Characteristics

- Rate: atrial rate 250–350 bpm, ventricular rate slower, usually 100–150 bpm
- Ventricular rhythm: usually regular, may be irregular
- P waves: typical sawtooth pattern
- PR interval: may be unable to determine
- P wave/QRS relationship: some relationship is present; each QRS complex is associated with a P wave, but many nonconducted P waves are present
- Extra or abnormal beats: none except for nonconducted P waves

Treatment

- If ventricular response is >100 bpm and patient has hypotension, decreased level of consciousness, chest pain, pale or diaphoretic skin, treatment includes:
  –Administer oxygen.
  –Obtain venous access.
  –Administer **digitalis** 0.25–0.5 mg IV if patient is **not** hypokalemic or **does not have** digitalis toxicity.
  –Consider administration of β-**blocker, verapamil, procainamide,** or **quinidine.**
  –Consider synchronized cardioversion if medications fail to convert rhythm.

Atrial Fibrillation

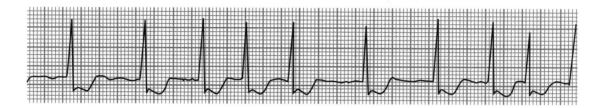

Characteristics

- Rate: atrial rate often >400 bpm, ventricular rate variable
- Ventricular rhythm: always irregular
- P waves: unable to determine configuration, underlying baseline is fine fibrillating waves
- PR interval: unable to determine
- P wave/QRS relationship: unable to determine
- QRS complex shape and width: usually of uniform shape and between 0.08 and 0.1 seconds in duration
- Extra or abnormal beats: none

Treatment

- If ventricular response is >100 bpm and the patient has hypotension, decreased level of consciousness, pale and diaphoretic skin, treatment includes:
  –Administer oxygen.
  –Obtain venous access.
  –Administer **digitalis** 0.25–0.5 mg IV if patient is **not** hypokalemic or **does not have** digitalis toxicity.
  –Consider administration of **verapamil, propranolol, procainamide,** or **quinidine.**
  –Consider synchronized cardioversion if medication fails to convert or slow rhythm.

First Degree Heart Block

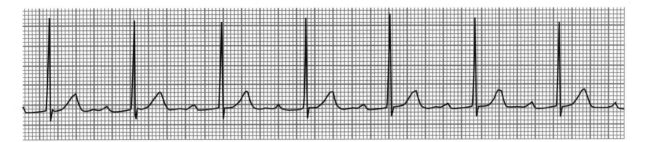

Characteristics

- Rate: usually 60–100 bpm
- Ventricular rhythm: regular
- P waves: present and uniformly shaped
- PR interval: >0.2 seconds
- P waves/QRS relationship: P wave associated with each QRS complex
- QRS complex shape and width: uniformly shaped and between 0.08–0.1 seconds in duration
- Extra or abnormal beats: none

Treatment

- Treat underlying cause if possible. If patient has hypotension, decreased level of consciousness, chest pain, pale and diaphoretic skin caused by slow ventricular response, treatment includes:
  - Administer 100% oxygen.
  - Obtain venous access.
  - Administer **atropine** 0.5–1 mg IV and repeat q3–5min up to a maximum dose of 0.04 mg/kg.
  - Apply transcutaneous (external) cardiac pacing.
  - Administer **dopamine** 5–10 µg/kg/min IV infusion.
  - Administer **epinephrine** 2–10 µg/min IV infusion.
  - Administer **isoproterenol** IV infusion at low dose.
  - Consider transvenous cardiac pacing.

Second Degree Heart Block: Mobitz Type I

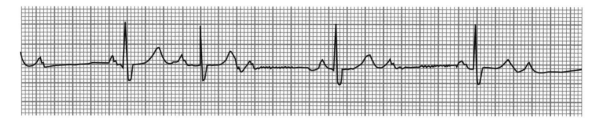

Characteristics

- Rate: usually between 60 and 100 bpm, atrial rate is higher than ventricular rate because of nonconducted sinus impulses
- Ventricular rhythm: irregular
- P waves: present and uniformly shaped
- PR interval: varying duration, cycle begins with an interval between 0.12 and 0.2 seconds; the interval gradually lengthens until blocked ventricular conduction occurs; the interval then reverts to 0.12 to 0.2 seconds, and gradual lengthening of the interval again occurs
- P wave/QRS relationship: each QRS complex has an associated P wave; however, P waves occur with no associated QRS complex because of blocked conduction
- QRS complex shape and width: uniformly shaped and between 0.08 and 0.1 seconds in duration
- Extra or abnormal beats: none except for nonconducted P waves

Treatment

- Frequently no treatment is required unless patient has hypotension, decreased level of consciousness, pale and diaphoretic skin, or chest pain caused by a slow ventricular response. Treatment then includes:
–Administer 100% oxygen.
–Obtain venous access.
–Administer **atropine** 0.5–1 mg IV and repeat q3–5min up to a maximum dose of 0.04 mg/kg.
–Apply transcutaneous (external) cardiac pacing.
–Administer **dopamine** 5–10 μg/kg/min IV infusion.
–Administer **epinephrine** 2–10 μg/min IV infusion.
–Administer **isoproterenol** IV infusion at low dose.
–Consider transvenous cardiac pacing.

Second Degree Heart Block: Mobitz Type II

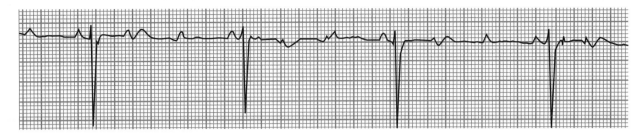

Characteristics

- Rate: atrial rate usually between 60 and 100 bpm, ventricular rate is slower, often between 40 and 60 bpm
- Ventricular rhythm: usually regular but may be irregular
- P waves: present and uniformly shaped
- PR interval: usually between 0.12 and 0.2 seconds but may be prolonged; interval remains constant when ventricular conduction occurs
- P wave/QRS relationship: each QRS complex is preceeded by two or more P waves; not all P waves are conducted
- QRS complex shape and width: uniformly shaped and usually between 0.08 and 0.1 seconds in duration; duration may be >0.1 seconds because of conduction system defects
- Extra or abnormal beats: none except for nonconducted P waves

Treatment

- Treatment is directed toward improving the ventricular rate and cardiac output. If the patient has hypotension, decreased level of consciousness, pale and diaphoretic skin, or chest pain, treatment includes:
  –Administer 100% oxygen.
  –Obtain venous access.
  –Administer **atropine** 0.5–1 mg IV and repeat q3–5min up to a maximum dose of 0.04 mg/kg.
  –Apply transcutaneous (external) cardiac pacing.
  –Administer **dopamine** 5–10 µg/kg/min IV infusion.
  –Administer **epinephrine** 2–10 µg/min IV infusion.
  –Administer **isoproterenol** IV infusion at low doses.
  –Consider transvenous cardiac pacing.

Third Degree Heart Block

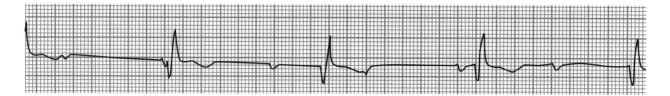

Characteristics

- Rate: atrial rate usually between 60 and 100 bpm, ventricular rate usually between 20 and 40 bpm
- Ventricular rhythm: regular, may be irregular if escape beats occur
- P waves: present and uniformly shaped
- PR interval: varying duration
- P wave/QRS relationship: none, atrial contraction and ventricular contraction are independent of each other
- QRS complex shape and width: uniformly shaped, unless escape beats originate from a different ventricular or nodal foci; QRS width is usually >0.12 seconds
- Extra or abnormal beats: usually none; however, junctional or ventricular escape beats may appear

Treatment

- Administer 100% oxygen.
- Obtain venous access.
- Administer **atropine** 0.5–1 mg IV and repeat q3–5min up to a maximum dose of 0.04 mg/kg.
- Apply transcutaneous (external) cardiac pacing.
- Administer **dopamine** 5–10 µg/kg/min IV infusion.
- Administer **epinephrine** 2–10 µg/min IV infusion.
- Administer **isoproterenol** IV infusion at a low dose.
- Consider transvenous cardiac pacing.

Premature Ventricular Contractions (PVCs)

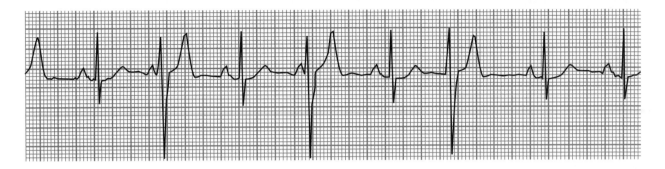

Characteristics

- Rate: usually 60–100 bpm
- Ventricular rhythm: irregular because of premature beats, but the premature beats may occur at regular intervals throughout the cycle; compensatory pause is present with the PVC
- P waves: present and uniformly shaped with each regular sinus initiated complex, not present with the PVC
- PR interval: between 0.12 and 0.2 seconds with each regular sinus initiated complex, not present with the PVC
- P wave/QRS complex relationship: a P wave is associated with each regular sinus initiated QRS complex, no P wave precedes the PVC
- QRS complex shape and width: each regular sinus initiated QRS complex is uniform in shape and between 0.08 and 0.1 seconds in duration; PVC complex(es) may be uniform or multiform in shape, and is (are) >0.12 seconds in duration
- Extra or abnormal beats: present, may occur in slow sinus rhythms

Treatment

- Directed toward suppressing PVCs and increasing cardiac output. PVCs that require treatment are (1) more than six PVCs occurring in 1 minute, (2) multiformed PVCs, (3) more than three consecutive PVCs, (4) PVCs appearing after MI, (5) PVCs entering the rhythm cycle near the preceding T wave, and (6) PVCs accompanied by chest pain. Treatment includes:
  –Administer oxygen.
  –Obtain venous access.
  –Correct electrolyte abnormalities if present (hypokalemia or hypomagnesemia).
  –Administer **lidocaine** 1–1.5 mg/kg IV with repeat dose of 0.5–0.75 mg/kg q5–10min, to maximum of 3 mg/kg if necessary; followed by continuous IV infusion of 2 g in 500 mL D5W at a 1–4 mg/min rate.
  –Administer **procainamide** 10–15 mg/kg IV at 20–30 mg/min, repeat the dosage until ectopy is suppressed or the maximum dose of 17 mg/kg is administered.
  –Administer **bretylium tosylate** 5 mg/kg IV followed by continuous IV infusion, 500 mg in 50 mL D5W, at a 1–2 mg/min rate.

Ventricular Tachycardia

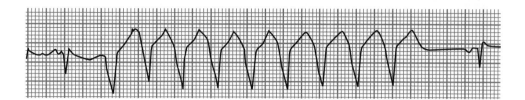

Characteristics

- Rate: 100–250 bpm
- Ventricular rhythm: regular
- P waves: none present
- PR interval: none present
- P wave/QRS complex relationship: none because of absence of P waves
- QRS complex shape and width: uniformly bizarre in shape, >0.12 seconds in duration
- Extra or abnormal beats: present

Treatment

Pulse Present

- Administer oxygen.
- Obtain venous access.
- Administer **lidocaine** 1–1.5 mg/kg IV then 0.5–0.75 mg/kg q5–10min until ectopy is suppressed or maximum dose of 3 mg/kg is administered.
- Administer **procainamide** 20–30 mg/min IV until ectopy is suppressed or maximum dose of 17 mg/kg is administered.
- If ectopy is still present, administer **bretylium** 5–10 mg/kg IV to ectopy suppression or maximum dose of 30 mg/kg.
- Synchronized cardioversion at 100, 200, 300, 360 J.

Pulseless

- Administer 100% oxygen and initiate CPR (precordial thump if witnessed).
- Defibrillate with 200 J.
- Defibrillate with 200–300 J.
- Continue CPR, assist with intubation.
- Obtain venous access.
- Administer 1 mg **epinephrine** IV, repeat q3–5min.
- Defibrillate with 360 J.
- Administer other medications such as **lidocaine, bretylium, magnesium sulfate, procainamide,** or **sodium bicarbonate.**
- Defibrillate with 360 J following each dose of medication.

Ventricular Fibrillation

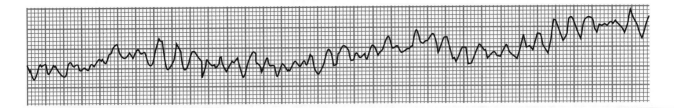

Characteristics

- Rate: undeterminable
- Ventricular rhythm: chaotic, irregular
- P waves: none present, no electrical stimulus occurring in the sinus node or atria
- PR interval: none present
- P waves/QRS relationship: none
- QRS complex shape and width: none present, undulation of baseline occurs
- Extra or abnormal beats: none

Treatment

- Administer 100% oxygen and initiate CPR.
- Defibrillate with 200 J.
- Defibrillate with 200–300, 360 J.
- Continue CPR and assist with intubation.
- Obtain venous access.
- Administer 1 mg **epinephrine** IV, repeat q3–5min.
- Defibrillate with 360 J.
- Administer other medications such as **lidocaine, bretylium, magnesium sulfate, procainamide,** or **sodium bicarbonate**.
- Defibrillate with 360 J following each dose of medication.

Asystole

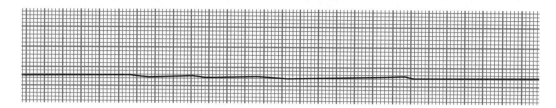

Characteristics

- Rate: none
- Ventricular rhythm: none
- P waves: none
- PR interval: none
- P wave/QRS relationship: none
- QRS complex shape and width: none
- Extra or abnormal beats: none

Treatment

- Administer 100% oxygen.
- Initiate CPR.
- Assist with intubation
- Obtain venous access.
- Consider and treat possible causes (hypoxia, hyperkalemia, hypokalemia, hypothermia, acidosis, drug overdose).
- Consider immediate transcutaneous (external) cardiac pacing.
- Administer **epinephrine** 1:10,000 1 mg IV, repeat q3–5min (in pediatric cardiac arrest, higher doses of epinephrine may be used). If unable to establish venous access, medication may be administered via endotracheal tube.
- Administer **atropine** 1 mg IV, repeat q3–5min to a maximum dosage of 0.04 mg/kg. If unable to establish venous access, medication may be administered via endotracheal tube.
- Consider administration of **sodium bicarbonate** 1 mEq/kg IV.

Appendicitis

Etiology
- Obstruction or infection of the appendix

Nursing Diagnoses
- Pain
- Infection

Common Complaints
- Abdominal pain eventually localizing in the right lower quadrant, anorexia, vomiting, diarrhea, fever; steady, progressive, localized pain lasting >6 hours with associated rebound tenderness and guarding suggests an emergent condition

Triage Rating
- Urgent

Related Factors
- Most common occurrence is in individuals between the ages of 10–30 years. While the appendix is most commonly located in the right lower quadrant, it may be flipped into the retrocecal space. In children <2 years of age, the pain associated with appendicitis is poorly localized, making diagnosis difficult, and perforation more likely. Obstetric patients with appendicitis are more prone to developing peritonitis, and subsequent mortality rates are approximately 20%. The majority of the time, the diagnosis of acute appendicitis is made by history.

Assessment Findings
- Low-grade fever
- Decreased bowel sounds
- Palpable pain over McBurney's point
- Rebound tenderness
- Positive Rovsing's sign (pressure applied to left lower quadrant intensifies right-sided pain)
- Positive psoas sign (hyperextension of right hip causes pain) and obturator sign (pain with flexion and internal rotation of right thigh) with perforation

Diagnostics
- CBC: WBC frequently elevated >10,000 but not always; possible presence of left shift
- Sedimentation rate: may be elevated
- Pregnancy test: should be performed on childbearing-aged girls and women
- Radiographic studies: abdominal film possibly indicating fecalith; pelvic ultrasound possibly indicating free fluid or abscess or other pathology; CT scan possibly demonstrating abscess or other pathology

Interventions
- Place patient in position of comfort.
- Insert IV and infuse fluids of NS or D5.45 NS.
- Obtain blood samples for CBC, chemistries, and other laboratory studies.
- Insert nasogastric tube and attach to suction.
- Administer antibiotic medications:
  –**Ticarcillin-clavulanate** 3.1 g IV infusion *or* **cefoxitin** 2 g IV infusion *and* **metronidazole** 500 mg IV infusion.
- Administer pain relief medications:
  –**Meperidine** 25–100 mg IV/IM.
- Monitor temperature, BP, pulse rate and rhythm, respiratory rate, pain relief, urinary output.

Disposition If perforation has occurred or there is a high suspicion of acute appendicitis, admission to the operating suite is required. Otherwise, observe for 4–6 hours or release to home with instructions to return in 4–6 hours for a second set of laboratory studies or sooner if pain increases.

Bowel Obstruction/Intussusception

Etiology
- Adhesions, tumors, gallstones, fecal impaction, hernia, paralytic ileus, or intussusception

Nursing Diagnoses
- Pain
- Altered tissue perfusion: bowel
- Risk for fluid volume deficit
- Risk for infection

Common Complaints
- Abdominal pain, vomiting, constipation, or diarrhea. Steady, progressive, localized pain >6 hours with rebound tenderness and guarding suggests an emergent condition. In children with intussusception, sudden acute colicky abdominal pain may be present along with bloody stools (like currant jelly).

Triage Rating
- Urgent to emergent

Related Factors
- Obstructions can occur in either the small or large intestines. As the abdomen distends, the blood supply to the bowel and absorption of fluid and electrolytes are both decreased. In children <2 years of age, obstruction may be caused by intussusception, volvulus, Hirschsprung's disease, or strangulated hernias. Complications include sepsis and hypovolemia, both of which increase the mortality rate.

Assessment Findings
- Abdominal distension
- Possible abdominal scars from previous surgery
- Hyperactive or hypoactive bowel sounds
- Tympanic percussion sounds over the abdomen
- Possible palpable obstruction mass in infants
- Tachycardia
- Hypotension

Diagnostics
- Radiographic studies: abdominal films demonstrating distended bowel loops with air fluid levels; barium enema possibly indicating level of obstruction
- CBC: elevated WBC possible because of infection; decreased hemoglobin and hematocrit possible from fluid volume loss
- Chemistries: possible electrolyte loss with vomiting and diarrhea
- ABG: metabolic acidosis (pH <7.35, HCO_3 <22 mm Hg) if significant dehydration is present

Interventions
- Place patient in position of comfort.
- Insert IV and infuse fluids of NS or consider D5.2 NS in pediatric patients.
- Obtain blood samples for CBC, chemistries, and other laboratory studies.
- Insert nasogastric tube and attach to suction.
- Consider administration of antibiotic medication:
  - **Cefoxitin** 1–2 g IV infusion.
- Consider administration of pain relief medication:
  - **Meperidine** 25–100 mg IM/IV.
- Monitor BP, pulse rate and rhythm, respiratory rate, pulse oximetry, nasogastric tube output, pain relief.

Disposition   Admission to hospital, possible operating suite for surgical decompression.

Cholecystitis

Etiology
- Stasis of bile in the gallbladder from duct obstruction

Nursing Diagnoses
- Pain
- Risk for infection

Common Complaints
- Colicky abdominal pain in right upper quadrant, referred pain to right shoulder or scapula, vomiting (often with improvement in pain following vomiting)

Triage Rating
- Urgent

Related Factors
- Gallstones are the usual cause of gallbladder or bile duct obstruction. Risk factors for gallstone formation include obesity, use of oral contraceptives, pregnancy, and genetic factors.

Assessment Findings
- Increased temperature
- Tachycardia
- Tachypnea
- Abdominal guarding with palpation
- Positive Murphy's sign (inability to breathe deeply during palpation of the gallbladder)

Diagnostics
- Radiographic studies: ultrasound may demonstrate the presence of gallstones or thickened gallbladder wall
- CBC: elevated WBC possible if condition is caused by infection
- Chemistries: altered electrolytes possible if persistent vomiting has occurred

Interventions
- Place patient in position of comfort.
- Insert IV and infuse NS fluid.
- Obtain blood samples for CBC, chemistries, and other laboratory studies.
- Insert nasogastric tube and attach to suction.
- Administer antiemetic medication:
  –**Prochlorperazine** 5–10 mg IV *or* **promethazine** 25 mg IM.
- Administer pain relief medication:
  –**Meperidine** 25–100 mg IM/IV.
- Monitor BP, pulse rate and rhythm, respiratory rate, pulse oximetry, nasogastric tube output, pain relief.

Disposition   If vomiting and pain cannot be controlled with ED treatment, hospital admission is required. Otherwise the patient may be released to home with follow-up in 24–48 hours.

Diverticulitis

Etiology
- Fecalith, bacterial organism

Nursing Diagnoses
- Pain
- Risk for infection

Common Complaints
- Crampy abdominal pain located in the left lower quadrant, diarrhea or constipation, nausea, vomiting, fever

Triage Rating
- Nonurgent to urgent

Related Factors
- Most common in adults >50 years. The development of pouches, especially in the sigmoid colon, leads to the entrapment of fecal debris. Infection development can lead to abscess formation and perforation.

Assessment Findings
- Increased temperature
- Possible slight abdominal distension
- Normal or decreased bowel sounds
- Pain and possible guarding with abdominal palpation especially in the lower left quadrant

Diagnostics
- CBC: WBC elevated because of infection
- Chemistries: may be altered if prolonged vomiting or diarrhea has occurred
- Stool guaiac: positive for blood
- Radiologic studies: abdominal film demonstrating free air if perforation had occurred; abdominal ultrasound revealing inflammatory mass or abscess

Interventions
- Place patient in position of comfort.
- Insert IV and infuse NS fluid.
- Obtain blood sample for CBC, chemistries.
- Consider insertion of nasogastric tube and attach to suction.
- Administer antibiotic medications:
  –Mild infection: **Trimethoprim-sulfamethoxazole** 160/800 mg PO *or* **metronidazole** 500 mg PO.
  –Moderate/severe infection: **Cefoxitin** 1–2 g IV infusion *or* **gentamicin** 2 mg/kg IV infusion *and* **clindamycin** 300–900 mg IV infusion.
- Monitor BP, pulse rate and rhythm, respiratory rate, pulse oximetry, nasogastric tube output, pain relief.

Disposition   Individuals with mild infection can be released to home with instructions to increase fluids and fiber in diet. Stool softeners may be prescribed if constipation is present. Individuals with moderate to severe infections require hospital admission and possible surgical intervention.

Gastritis/Gastroenteritis

Etiology
- Ingested irritants, bacterial or viral organism, emotional stress

Nursing Diagnoses
- Pain
- Risk for fluid volume deficit
- Risk for infection

Common Complaints
- Diffuse abdominal pain, vomiting, possible diarrhea

Triage Rating
- Nonurgent

Related Factors
- The term *gastritis* relates to an inflammation of the stomach lining and involves the symptom of vomiting. The term *gastroenteritis* refers to an inflammation of both the gastric and intestinal mucosa. The inflammation is usually self-limiting without sequelae.

Assessment Findings
- Possible orthostatic changes
- Increased bowel sounds
- Diffuse abdominal tenderness with palpation without rebound or guarding
- Pediatric findings associated with dehydration:
  - Sunken fontanelle
  - Sunken eyes
  - Decreased tearing
  - Decreased urine output
  - Soft, doughy skin
  - Behavioral changes

Diagnostics
- Stool culture: may isolate offending organism*
- CBC: normal
- Chemistries: may be altered if prolonged vomiting or diarrhea has occurred

Interventions
- Place patient in position of comfort.
- Insert IV and infuse NS fluid if orthostatic changes are present.
- Obtain blood samples for CBC, chemistries.
- Administer antiemetic medication:
  - **Promethazine** 25–50 mg IM/PR (Peds: 1 mg/kg) *or* **prochlorperazine** 5–10 mg IV/IM, 25 mg PR (Peds: 0.13 mg/kg) *or* **trimethobenzamide** 200 mg IM/PR (Peds: 100–200 mg).
- Monitor BP, pulse rate and rhythm, respiratory rate, pain relief, vomiting episodes.

*If shigellosis is suspected, oral **trimethoprim-sulfamethoxazole** may be administered to shorten course.

Disposition
Release to home unless significant dehydration had occurred. Home instructions include:

Pediatric oral rehydration

For diarrhea:
- <2 years give ½ cup of oral electolyte solution (do not use fluids such as sport drinks, cola drinks, or apple juice, as these can worsen diarrhea caused by sugar) every hour using a small spoon.
- >2 years give ½ to 1 cup of oral electrolyte solution (do not use fluids such as sport drinks, cola drinks, or apple juice, as these can worsen diarrhea caused by sugar) every hour.
- Continue to feed child: if breast-fed, continue to breast-feed; if receiving formula, continue to give formula; if on solid foods, continue to give regular diet.

For vomiting:
- Give 1 teaspoon of oral electrolyte solution q2–3min until vomiting stops.

Adult oral rehydration

- Clear liquids only until 8–12 hours have passed without vomiting. Ingest 1 tablespoon q10min. If vomiting does not occur, double the amount each hour. If vomiting continues, wait 2–3 hours then start again with 1 tablespoon.
- Begin bland foods following 8–12 hours without vomiting and gradually resume normal diet.
- Diarrhea may also be treated with **loperamide** 4 mg PO or **attapulgite** 30 mL PO after each loose stool.

Gastrointestinal Bleeding

Etiology
- Esophageal varices, ulcerations, tumor, corrosive ingestion, Mallory-Weiss tear, foreign body ingestion with laceration, diverticulitis, colitis, injury

Nursing Diagnoses
- Fluid volume deficit
- Altered tissue perfusion

Common Complaints
- Bloody vomitus or stool, lightheadedness, diaphoresis, weakness, syncope

Triage Rating
- Urgent to emergent

Related Factors
- Chronic alcohol ingestion is associated with esophageal varices, whereas acute alcohol ingestion may cause a Mallory-Weiss tear. Ulcer disease may result from ingestion of medications such as aspirin or other NSAIDs. Ulcer formation has also been associated with genetic predisposition, infection, diet, stress, and smoking. The incidence of colorectal malignancy increases in persons >50 years.

Assessment Findings
- Restlessness or decreased level of consciousness
- Hypotension
- Tachycardia
- Pale, diaphoretic skin
- Blood in vomitus or stool
- Possible abdominal tenderness with palpation
- Normal, hyperactive, or hypoactive bowel sounds

Diagnostics
- Hemoccult slide: positive for blood in stomach contents or stool
- CBC: possible decreased hemoglobin and hematocrit
- Radiographic studies: chest film possibly identifying areas of obstruction or mediastinal air if perforation has occurred

Interventions
- Administer oxygen 6–15 L via face mask.
- Insert IV and infuse NS fluid.
- Obtain blood samples for CBC, chemistries, PT and PTT studies, and type and crossmatch.
- Insert nasogastric tube and attach to suction.
- Insert indwelling urinary catheter.
- If moderate to severe upper gastrointestinal tract bleeding, perform gastric lavage with room temperature NS fluid.
- Monitor level of consciousness, BP, pulse rate and rhythm, respiratory rate, pulse oximetry, nasogastric tube output, urinary output, amount of active bleeding.

Disposition   If moderate to severe bleeding, hospital admission is required. Individuals with mild bleeding that is controlled with ED treatment may be released to home with follow-up within 24 hours.

Pancreatitis

Etiology
- Injury, obstruction, alcohol or medication toxicity or ingestion, bacterial or viral infection

Nursing Diagnoses
- Pain
- Risk for fluid volume deficit
- Risk for impaired gas exchange

Common Complaints
- Extreme epigastric pain that radiates to the back; vomiting, diaphoresis, dyspnea

Triage Rating
- Urgent

Related Factors
- Autodigestion of the pancreas by its own enzymes is caused by various factors. Fifty percent of patients with pancreatitis have associated cholelithiasis,. Twenty-five percent have a history of chronic alcohol abuse, and 10% have had a direct injury to the area. Pleural effusion and atelectasis are often present in the acute stages. Children can develop pancreatitis from toxic medication ingestion, but alcohol ingestion must also be considered. Pregnant women are also at risk from the formation of gallstones.

Assessment Findings
- Restlessness
- Hypotension
- Tachycardia
- Tachypnea with decreased breath sounds in the bases and possible rales/rhonchi
- Pale, diaphoretic skin
- Possible increased temperature
- Abdominal distension
- Decreased bowel sounds
- Abdominal tenderness with possible rebound, guarding, and rigidity
- Discoloration around the umbilicus indicates hemorrhage

Diagnostics
- CBC: elevated WBC because of injury or inflammation
- Chemistry: elevated amylase, elevated glucose
- Lipase: elevated
- Liver enzymes: possibly elevated from alcohol use
- Urine: elevated amylase
- Radiographic studies: chest film possibly demonstrating pleural effusion or atelectasis along with elevated diaphragm; ultrasound possibly identifying duct obstruction from stone formation

Interventions
- Place patient in position of comfort.
- Insert IV and infuse NS fluid.
- Obtain blood samples for CBC, amylase, lipase, chemistries, and other studies.
- Insert nasogastric tube and attach to suction if vomiting is present.
- Administer pain relief medications:
  – **Meperidine** 25–100 mg IV.
- Consider administration of antispasmodic medication if bowel function is present:
  – **Dicyclomine** 20 mg IM *or* **propantheline bromide** 15 mg PO for mild episodes.
- Monitor level of consciousness, BP, pulse rate and rhythm, respiratory rate, pulse oximetry, nasogastric tube output, pain relief.

Disposition   Hospital admission is required for pain management and continued monitoring.

Pyloric Stenosis

Etiology
- Anatomic narrowing of the pyloric opening

Nursing Diagnoses
- Altered tissue perfusion: bowel
- Risk for fluid volume deficit

Common Complaints
- Forceful or projectile vomiting, lethargy, failure to thrive

Triage Rating
- Urgent

Related Factors
- Occurs most commonly in first born sons within the first month of life. The passage of ingestant is difficult because of the narrowed opening between the distal end of the stomach and the duodenum.

Assessment Findings
- Minimal weight gain from birth or actual weight loss
- Tachycardia
- Palpable "olive shaped" mass at pylorus

Diagnostics
- Radiographic studies: abdominal film possibly demonstrating gastric dilation; ultrasound indicating obstruction; barium swallow revealing a "string sign" and delayed gastric emptying
- Chemistries: altered electrolytes possible because of poor nutrition and electrolyte loss

Interventions
- Insert IV and infuse D5.25 NS fluid.
- Obtain blood samples for CBC, chemistries, and other studies.
- Monitor pulse rate and rhythm, respiratory rate, and episodes of emesis.

Disposition   Admission to the operating suite for surgical repair of the stenosis.

Ulcer

Etiology
- Bacterial organisms, HIV, stress, eroding medications

Nursing Diagnoses
- Pain
- Risk for infection

Common Complaints
- Burning, gnawing pain in the epigastric area that may radiate to the back; pain may be associated with food intake; nausea and vomiting

Triage Rating
- Urgent

Related Factors
- Ulceration of the gastric mucosa leads to excoriation and mucous membrane sloughing. An imbalance between pepsin, hydrochloric acid secretion and bicarbonate causes gastric erosion. Bacteria invasion from *Helicobacter pylori* has been implicated as a causative factor. Chronic ingestion of gastric mucosa irritating medication such as aspirin or nonsteroidal antiinflammatory drugs (NSAIDs) can also lead to the development of ulcers. Ulcers occur most commonly in individuals ages 20–60 years but can occur in children. During pregnancy, women with previous ulcer disease may experience improvement in symptoms.

Assessment Findings
- Possible positive orthostatic changes
- Decreased bowel sounds
- Pain with palpation over mid-epigastric area
- Possible guarding with palpation

Diagnostics
- CBC: elevated WBC if bacterial infection present; decreased hemoglobin and hematocrit if bleeding has or is presently occurring
- Hemoccult slide: stomach contents or stool may be positive for blood
- Radiographic studies: abdominal films demonstrating free air if perforation has occurred

Interventions
- Place patient in position of comfort.
- Insert IV and infuse NS fluids if positive orthostatic vital signs.
- Obtain blood samples for CBC, chemistries, and other studies.
- Insert nasogastric tube and attach to suction if vomiting present.
- Perform gastric lavage with NS fluid if blood present in stomach contents.
- Administer antacid medications:
  –**Magnesium** or **aluminum hydroxide** 30 mL **hyoscyamine sulfate (Donnatal elixir)** 10–15 mL, *and* **lidocaine (Viscous Xylocaine)** 5 mL PO.
  –**Cimetidine** 300 mg PO or IV infusion *or* **ranitidine** 150 mg PO or 50 mg IV.
- Monitor BP, pulse rate and rhythm, respiratory rate, pulse oximetry, nasogastric tube output, pain relief.

Disposition   Admission to hospital if bleeding is present. If no bleeding is present, patient may be released to home with follow-up in 24–48 hours and dietary instruction:
- Small, nutritious, regularly scheduled meals
- Avoid irritating substances such as caffeine, alcohol, foods that precipitate symptoms, and irritating medications

Unit VII

Genitourinary-Gynecologic Conditions

Epididymitis

Etiology
- Bacterial, enteric organisms, vesicoureteral reflux

Nursing Diagnoses
- Pain
- Risk for infection

Common Complaints
- Scrotal pain that may radiate into groin, fever, possible urinary frequency and dysuria

Triage Rating
- Urgent

Related Factors
- Commonly associated with sexually transmitted diseases or prostatic infection. The infection is usually unilateral but may be bilateral. Rare before the age of puberty.

Assessment Findings
- Increased temperature
- Tachycardia
- "Duck waddle" walk
- Swollen red scrotum
- Tender testes
- Pain relief with scrotal elevation

Diagnostics
- Urinalysis: >3–5 WBC/hpf, >0–2 RBC/hpf, positive nitrate or bacteriuria
- CBC: possible elevated WBC with a left shift
- Radiographic studies: radionuclide scan of the scrotum to determine if torsion is present

Interventions
- Elevate affected scrotum.
- Apply intermittent ice pack to scrotal area.
- Administer antibiotic medications:
  - <35 years of age:
  - **Ceftriaxone** 250–500 mg IM *and* **tetracycline** 500 mg PO qid *or* **doxycycline** 100 mg PO bid.
  - >35 years of age:
  - **Trimethoprim-sulfamethoxazole** PO bid.
- Monitor temperature, BP, pulse rate and rhythm, pain relief.

Disposition   Release to home with instruction for follow-up in 7–10 days and abstinence from intercourse.

Penile Injury

Etiology
- Blunt or penetrating forces, foreign objects, zippers, bites

Nursing Diagnoses
- Pain
- Risk for infection

Common Complaints
- Pain of the genital area, skin abrasions, blood in the urine

Triage Rating
- Urgent

Related Factors
- Depending on the type of injury, either the testicle or the penis, or both, may be involved. Assessment findings and treatments will vary depending on the exact nature of the injury.

Assessment Findings
- Testicular injury: scrotal discoloration, swelling
- Foreskin entrapment: usually caused by a zipper, with observable skin caught in the zipper
- Bite: puncture wound on penile skin, swelling
- Penile fracture: flaccid penis, hematoma, penis deviated away from involved site
- Foreign object: hematuria, possible urinary retention, genital discharge, and edema

Diagnostics
- Urinalysis: may demonstrate presence of RBC
- Radiographic studies: may indicate presence of foreign object or urethral laceration with penile rupture or fracture; testicular ultrasound is effective in demonstrating rupture

Interventions
- Testicular injury: surgical decompression is necessary.
- Entrapment: apply mineral oil to zipper and attempt to release zipper from foreskin. If not effective, cut median bar of zipper to release locking mechanism. Sedation is often required.
- Bites: irrigate with NS and consider debridement. Administer antibiotic medication:
  –**Cefazolin** 1–2 g IV infusion (Peds: 25–100 mg/kg).
- Administer **dT** 0.5 mL IM if required.
- Foreign object: transurethral removal or possible surgical removal.

Disposition   If surgical intervention is necessary, the patient will require hospital admission. Otherwise, the patient may be released to home with close follow-up in 24 hours and instructions to return if symptoms indicating infection occur or the patient has difficulty urinating.

Priapism

Etiology
- Frequently unknown

Nursing Diagnoses
- Pain
- Altered tissue perfusion: penis

Common Complaints
- Painful penile erection, inability to urinate

Triage Rating
- Emergent

Related Factors
- Priapism is defined as a prolonged penile erection without sexual desire. The glans penis and corpus spongiosum are flaccid, with tenseness and congestion of the corpora cavernosa. Hematologic diseases such as sickle cell anemia, oncologic disorders, spinal cord injury, neurologic disorders, and infection have been identified with this disorder. Also, use of marijuana and ingestion of thioridazine, phenothiazines, anticoagulants, and guanethidine have been implicated with priapism.

Assessment Findings
- Tenseness of the corpora cavernosa with flaccidity of the glans penis and corpus spongiosum
- Tachycardia

Diagnostics
- None

Interventions
- Administer oxygen 6–15 L via face mask if sickle cell anemia is present.
- Insert IV or saline lock.
- Administer pain relief medication:
  - **Morphine sulfate** 2–10 mg IV *or* **meperidine** 25–100 mg IM/IV.
- Administer ice water enemas.
- Consider assistance with aspiration of blood from corpora cavernosa.
- Monitor pain relief, erection resolution, and urinary output.

Disposition   Hospital admission is required for patients with underlying disease or if priapism is not resolved in the ED.

Orchitis

Etiology
- Mumps, sexually transmitted organisms

Nursing Diagnoses
- Pain
- Infection

Common Complaints
- Fever, testicular pain radiating to groin

Triage Rating
- Urgent

Related Factors
- If associated with mumps, the onset of testicular inflammation usually occurs 3–10 days following the onset of parotitis. Orchitis is also commonly present with epididymitis.

Assessment Findings
- Possible increased temperature
- Enlarged scrotum with erythema and edema

Diagnostics
- Urinalysis: may indicate elevated bacteria or microhematuria
- Radiographic studies: ultrasound possibly identifying scrotal mass, torsion, or rupture

Interventions
- Elevate affected scrotum.
- Administer antibiotic medication if not mumps related:
  –**Ceftriaxone** 250–500 g IM *and* **tetracycline** 500 mg PO.
- Assist with possible infiltration of plain lidocaine into spermatic cord to decrease pain.
- Monitor temperature, BP, pulse rate and rhythm, pain relief.

Disposition   Release to home with follow-up in 2–3 days.

Testicular Torsion

Etiology
- Unknown or possible injury

Nursing Diagnoses
- Pain
- Altered tissue perfusion: testis

Common Complaints
- Testicular pain with sudden onset, nausea/vomiting

Triage Rating
- Emergent

Related Factors
- Commonly occurs at the age of puberty but may occur in men >21 years of age. This is responsible for approximately 40% of the cases of acute scrotal swelling and pain. Torsion occurs from a rotation of the testis on the spermatic cord, causing a compromise of the blood supply. Necrosis of the testis will result if the torsion is not relieved within 4–6 hours.

Assessment Findings
- Tachycardia
- Erythema, edema, and tautness of affected scrotal skin
- Possible unequal height of testes
- Tender and abnormal position of epididymis
- Absent cremasteric reflex

Diagnostics
- CBC: no elevation of WBC
- Urinalysis: normal findings
- Radiographic studies: Doppler ultrasound indicating absent or decreased artery pulsations; radionuclide imaging of the scrotum demonstrating decreased perfusion

Interventions
- Insert IV or saline lock.
- Administer pain relief medication:
  - **Meperidine** 25–100 mg IM/IV.
  - **Morphine sulfate** 2–10 mg IM/IV.
- Assist with possible manual release of torsion using cord block anesthesia.
- Monitor BP, pulse rate and rhythm, episodes of emesis, pain relief.

Disposition
Hospital admission to operating suite for surgical correction if manual manipulation is not successful in restoring blood flow.

Ovarian Cyst

Etiology
- Normal hormonal cycle, neoplasm, or overgrowth of endometrial tissue

Nursing Diagnoses
- Pain

Common Complaints
- Abdominal pain diffuse or localized, nausea/vomiting

Triage Rating
- Urgent

Related Factors
- The pain associated with an ovarian cyst most frequently occurs during the last half of the regular menstrual cycle, or menses cycle may be irregular. The pain may range from mild to severe. Women who use oral contraceptives are less likely to develop ovarian cysts. Vomiting has been associated as an early symptom of torsion.

Assessment Findings
- Tachycardia
- Palpable abdominal pain and possible guarding
- Pelvic examination: adnexal tenderness

Diagnostics
- CBC: no elevation of WBC
- Radiographic studies: pelvic ultrasound identifies the majority of cysts
- Pregnancy test: negative
- Possible culdocentesis: fluid or serosanguineous fluid may be aspirated

Interventions
- Place patient in a position of comfort.
- Insert IV and infuse NS fluids.
- Administer pain relief medications:
  - **Meperidine** 25–100 mg IM/IV.
- Monitor BP, pulse rate and rhythm, pain relief.

Disposition   Hospital admission may be required for further diagnostic tests such as laparoscopy. If pain relief is obtained with ED treatment, patient may be released to home with close follow-up in 1–2 days.

Pelvic Inflammatory Disease (PID)

Etiology
- Bacterial organisms including *Neisseria*

Nursing Diagnoses
- Pain
- Infection

Common Complaints
- Lower abdominal pain, vaginal discharge, spotting between menstrual periods, fever

Triage Rating
- Urgent

Related Factors
- Common organisms include *Neisseria gonorrhoeae*, or *Chlamydia trachomatis*. This is frequently a polymicrobial infection. The infection begins as a cervicitis and if untreated progresses to endometritis and salpingitis. Associated risk factors include adolescence, multiple sexual partners, previous episodes of sexually transmitted diseases, and intrauterine devices to prevent pregnancy. Currently the highest rate of PID is found in the age group of 15–19 years.

Assessment Findings
- Possible increased temperature
- Tachycardia
- "Shuffle" gait
- Abdominal tenderness to palpation with possible guarding and rebound
- Pelvic examination:
  - Cervical inflammation
  - Mucopurulent discharge
  - Cervical motion tenderness
  - Possible adnexal masses or abscess or uterine tenderness

Diagnostics
- Pregnancy test: ectopic pregnancy possible cause of symptoms
- Urinalysis: if bacteria present, urine infection may be cause of symptoms
- Wet mount of vaginal discharge: if number of WBCs hpf is less than number of epithelial cells, PID not present; may also indicate presence of trichomonads
- Cervical cultures or gram stain: especially for *Chlamydia* infection and gonorrhea
- CBC: possible elevated WBC with left shift caused by infection
- Sedimentation rate: may be elevated
- VDRL: presence of concurrent syphilis
- Radiographic studies: pelvic ultrasound demonstrating ectopic pregnancy if present

Interventions
- Insert IV and infuse NS fluids.
- Obtain blood samples for CBC, sedimentation rate, VDRL, and other studies.
- Administer antibiotic medications:
  - **Cefoxitin** 2 g IM/IV infusion *and* **doxycycline** 100 mg PO *or* **ofloxacin** 400 mg PO *and* **metronidazole** 500 mg PO.
- Administer pain relief medication:
  - **Meperidine** 25–100 mg IM/IV.
- Monitor temperature, pulse rate and rhythm, BP, pain relief.

Disposition
If acutely ill, hospitalization is required for continuous IV antibiotic therapy. Otherwise, patient may be released to home with close follow-up within 72 hours. Instructions must include:
- Sexual partner(s) must be evaluated and treated.
- Abstain from sexual intercourse until infection is completely treated.
- Use barrier methods during sexual intercourse to prevent future disease.

Sexually Transmitted Diseases

Etiology
- Varies depending on offending organism

Nursing Diagnoses
- Pain
- Infection

Common Complaints/Findings
- *Neisseria gonorrhoeae*: yellow genital discharge; dysuria; gram stain indicates gram-negative intracellular diplococcus; positive Thayer-Martin culture
- *Chlamydia trachomatis:* mucopurulent vaginal discharge; urethral itching and white penile discharge; positive culture
- *Trichomonas vaginalis*: thin, frothy, greenish-gray foul discharge, vaginal itching; organisms present on NS wet mount
- *Gardnerella vaginalis*: thin, frothy, gray-white discharge with a fishy odor
- *Candida albicans:* vaginal itching, inflamed vulva or glans penis, thick white discharge; patient should be questioned about HIV and diabetes
- Herpes simplex II: painful genital vesicular lesions
- *Treponema pallidum*: genital ulcer or chancre; positive VDRL reactive test
- Condyloma acuminatum: vaginal or penile wart type lesions that may be in clusters and may bleed

Triage Rating
- Nonurgent

Related Factors
- The offending organism is transmitted through sexual activity with an infected partner. Treatment must be administered to the patient and the infected partner. Both persons must refrain from sexual activity until treatment is complete.

Organism	Incubation Period	Treatment
• *Neisseria gonorrhoeae*	• 3–5 days	• **Ceftriaxone** 1 g IM *or* **ofloxacin** 400 mg PO (1 dose)
• *Chlamydia trachomatis*	• 5–10 days	• **Doxycycline** 100 mg bid × 7 days *or* **azithromycin** 1 g PO (1 dose)
• *Trichomonas vaginalis*	• 1 week	• **Metronidazole** 2 g PO (1 dose) *or* **metronidazole** 500 mg tid × 7 days
• *Gardnerella vaginalis*	• 5–10 days	• **Metronidazole** 2 g PO (1 dose) *or* **metronidazole** 500 mg tid × 7 days
• *Candida albicans*	• Variable	• **Clotrimazole** 1% cream or tablet intravaginally or applied to glans penis × 7–14 days
• Herpes simplex II	• 2–12 days	• **Acyclovir** 200 mg 5 times/d × 7–10 days
• *Treponema pallidum*	• 3 weeks	• Primary: **benzathine penicillin G** 2–4 million units IM
		• Latent: **benzathine penicillin G** 7.2 million units IM given as 2.4 million U/wk × 3 weeks
• Condyloma acuminatum	• 5–10 days	• **Podofilox** 0.5% solution for self-treatment bid × 3 days

Pyelonephritis

Etiology
- Bacterial organism

Nursing Diagnoses
- Pain
- Infection
- Risk for fluid volume deficit

Common Complaints
- Fever, back pain, nausea/vomiting

Triage Rating
- Urgent

Related Factors
- This upper urinary tract infection is frequently the result of an ascending gram-negative organism, especially *Escherichia coli*. If pregnancy is also present, the risk of premature delivery in untreated pyelonephritis is increased. Prolonged vomiting can lead to dehydration.

Assessment Findings
- Increased temperature
- Tachycardia
- Tenderness with percussion of affected flank area

Diagnostics
- Urinalysis: increased WBC because of infection
- CBC: possible elevated WBC from infection

Interventions
- Insert IV and infuse NS fluid.
- Administer antiemetic medication:
  - **Promethazine** 25 mg IV/IM.
  - **Prochlorperazine** 5–10 mg IM/IV.
- Administer antibiotic medication:
  - Moderate to severe infection:
  - **Ampicillin** 1 g IV infusion (Peds: 200 mg/kg/d) *and* **gentamicin** 1.5 mg/kg IV infusion (Peds: 2.5 mg/kg).
  - Mild infection:
  - **Trimethoprim-sulfamethoxazole** PO *or* **norfloxacin** 400 mg PO *or* **amoxicillin** 500 mg PO.
- Monitor BP, pulse rate and rhythm, temperature, vomiting episodes, pain relief.

Disposition   The majority of patients with pyelonephritis require hospital admission, both for IV antibiotic treatment and correction of possible dehydration. Mild infections may be treated on an outpatient basis with close follow-up within 72 hours.

Renal Calculi

Etiology
- Unknown, although associated with calcium-rich diets

Nursing Diagnoses
- Pain
- Altered urinary elimination

Common Complaints
- Back, abdominal, groin pain; vomiting; sweating

Triage Rating
- Urgent

Related Factors
- The majority of renal stones are calcium based. Males are more commonly affected than females, with increased frequency in the United States geographic areas of southern California, southern Great Lakes area, and southeastern states. Predisposing factors include hypercalcemia, hyperabsorption or reabsorption failure of the kidneys, and renal tubular acidosis.

Assessment Findings
- Extreme restlessness
- Tachycardia
- Pale, diaphoretic skin
- Palpable CVA tenderness

Diagnostics
- Urinalysis: hematuria present
- Radiographic studies: IVP possibly indicating level of obstruction or ureteral dilation

Interventions
- Position patient in position of comfort.
- Insert IV and infuse NS fluid.
- Strain all urine output.
- Administer pain relief medications:
  - **Morphine sulfate** 5–20 mg IV titrated to pain relief.
  - **Meperidine** 25–100 mg IV titrated to pain relief.
  - **Ketorolac** 60 mg IM or 30 mg IV.
- Administer antiemetic medication as needed:
  - **Promethazine** 25 mg IV.
  - **Prochlorperazine** 5–10 mg IM/IV.
- Monitor BP, pulse rate and rhythm, vomiting episodes, pain relief.

Disposition   If pain or vomiting continues unrelieved, hospital admission is necessary. If pain relief is obtained with ED treatment, release patient to home with instructions to increase fluid intake, strain all urine, and follow-up with a urologist within 2–3 days.

Urinary Retention

Etiology
- Prostatic enlargement, urethral stricture, diabetes, medications, tumor, recent removal of indwelling urinary catheter

Nursing Diagnoses
- Pain
- Altered urinary elimination

Common Complaints
- Abdominal pain, inability to void normal amounts of urine

Triage Rating
- Urgent

Related Factors
- The most common cause of urinary retention in the male population is benign prostatic enlargement. Anticholinergic medications such as antihistamines can also lead to this condition.

Assessment Findings
- Tachycardia
- Dull percussion sounds over distended bladder
- Palpable distended bladder

Diagnostics
- Urinalysis: possibly demonstrating bacteria if UTI or prostatitis is present

Interventions
- Insert indwelling urinary catheter and empty bladder in 500–800 mL increments.
- Consider irrigation of bladder with NS if drainage flow is obstructed after insertion of catheter.
- Monitor BP, pulse rate and rhythm, urinary output, pain relief.

Disposition　　Release patient to home with indwelling catheter in place. Close follow-up within 24–48 hours should occur to determine cause of urinary obstruction.

Urinary Tract Infection (UTI)

Etiology
- Bacterial organisms

Nursing Diagnoses
- Pain
- Infection

Common Complaints
- Lower abdominal pain, fever, urinary frequency and pain, hematuria

Triage Rating
- Nonurgent

Related Factors
- This infection of the lower urinary tract is more common in females than males. The common organisms involved include *Escherichia coli, Staphylococcus saprophyticus, Proteus mirabilis, Klebsiella pneumoniae, Chlamydia trachomatis,* and *Candida albicans.* Factors that increase the risk of developing a UTI in females are pregnancy, increased sexual activity, and use of barrier methods of birth control such as a diaphragm or spermicide use. In males risk factors include homosexuality, noncircumcision, HIV, and enlarged prostate gland.

Assessment Findings
- Possible increased temperature
- Suprapubic tenderness with palpation

Diagnostics
- Urinalysis: presence of bacteria and possibly RBCs

Interventions
- Administer analgesic medication:
  –**Phenazopyridine** 100–200 mg PO.
- Administer antibiotic medication:
  –**Trimethoprim-sulfamethoxazole** 80/400 or 160/800 mg PO.

Disposition   Release to home with instructions for follow-up within 1 week. Current therapy guidelines suggest treatment is effective with a 3- to 5-day course of antibiotics.

Unit VIII

Pregnancy-Related Conditions

Ectopic Pregnancy

Etiology
- Abnormal implantation site of embryo

Nursing Diagnoses
- Pain
- Risk for fluid volume deficit
- Anticipatory grieving

Common Complaints
- Unilateral low abdominal pain, vaginal bleeding, dizziness

Triage Rating
- Urgent to emergent

Related Factors
- The majority of ectopic pregnancies occur in the fallopian tube. Risk factors that increase the chance of ectopic pregnancy include previous tubal surgery, PID, use of an intrauterine device, infertility, abnormal tubal structure, prior salpingitis, and previous ectopic pregnancies.

Assessment Findings
- Possible positive orthostatic findings
- Abdominal tenderness with possible rebound tenderness and guarding
- Pelvic examination:
  - Vaginal bleeding or spotting
  - No obvious fetal tissue in vault

Diagnostics
- CBC: hemoglobin and hematocrit may be normal or low
- Pregnancy test: may be weakly positive or may be negative
- Radiographic studies: ultrasound revealing no intrauterine pregnancy but tissue mass at ectopic site
- Culdocentesis: presence of non-clotting blood with aspiration

Interventions
- Insert IV and infuse NS or D5LR fluids.
- Obtain blood samples for CBC, serum pregnancy test, type and crossmatch, and Rh factor.
- Administer pain medication:
  - **Meperidine** 25–100 mg IM/IV.
- Monitor BP, pulse rate and rhythm, respiratory rate, pulse oximetry, pain relief, emotional status.

Disposition Admission to the operating suite for removal of the ectopic pregnancy.

Miscarriage

Etiology
- Unknown or can be related to fever, trauma

Nursing Diagnoses
- Pain
- Anticipatory grieving
- Risk for fluid volume deficit

Common Complaints
- Abdominal pain and cramping, vaginal bleeding, missed menstrual period

Triage Rating
- Urgent

Related Factors
- Termination of a pregnancy prior to the twentieth week is termed a miscarriage. Different definitions of miscarriage are:
  –Threatened: closed cervical os; pregnancy may continue.
  –Inevitable: open cervical os; pregnancy cannot continue.
  –Incomplete: cervical os is open with tissue present in cervix or vaginal vault; pregnancy cannot continue.
  –Complete: cervical os is closed; tissue has passed; pregnancy has ended.
  –Septic: open cervical os; tissue may have passed or be present in cervix or vaginal vault; pregnancy cannot continue.
  –Missed: cervical os closed; no tissue has passed; fetus has died in utero.

Assessment Findings
- Possible tachycardia
- Possible hypotension
- Possible increased temperature
- Presence or absence of fetal heart tones
- Pelvic examination:
  –Vaginal bleeding
  –Cervical os open or closed
  –Possible presence of tissue in cervix or vaginal vault

Diagnostics
- Pregnancy test: positive
- Radiographic studies: ultrasound demonstrating a viable or nonviable pregnancy

Interventions
- Insert IV or saline lock.
- Obtain blood samples for CBC, serum pregnancy test, and type/Rh of maternal blood.
- Administer medications:
  –**Rho(D) immune globulin** if mother is Rh negative and miscarriage is inevitable, complete, missed, or septic.
  –**Methylergonovine** 0.2 mg IM if complete.
- Monitor BP, pulse rate and rhythm, respiratory rate, pulse oximetry, vaginal bleeding, emotional status.

Disposition   Prepare patient for dilation and curettage if miscarriage is inevitable or incomplete. Surgical intervention may be required for septic miscarriage. A missed miscarriage may also require surgical intervention, or the mother may be allowed to naturally deliver the expired fetus. For the patient experiencing a threatening miscarriage, home instructions include:
- Avoid sexual intercourse until recheck by obstetrician.
- Use sanitary pads for vaginal bleeding.
- Rest.
- Obtain close follow-up with obstetrician within 24–48 hours or return to the ED if symptoms worsen.

Placenta Abruptio

Etiology
- Trauma or unknown

Nursing Diagnoses
- Pain
- Fluid volume deficit

Common Complaints
- Vaginal bleeding, pain

Triage Rating
- Emergent

Related Factors
- While the incidence of premature separation of the placenta from the uterine wall is less than 3%, it is responsible for >15% of perinatal deaths. Predisposing factors include PIH, multiple gestation, substance abuse, advanced maternal age, previous placenta previa, gestational diabetes, precipitous delivery, and a short umbilical cord. Traumatic injury can also lead to this condition.

Assessment Findings
- Tachycardia
- Hypotension
- Pale, diaphoretic skin
- Dark red vaginal blood
- Decreased fetal heart tones
- Rigid uterus

Diagnostics
- CBC: possible decrease in hemoglobin and hematocrit
- Platelet count: used as baseline study
- PT, PTT, and clotting studies: used as baseline study since DIC is a complication
- Radiographic studies: ultrasound study demonstrating placenta abruptio

Interventions
- Administer oxygen 6–15 L via face mask.
- Insert IV and infuse NS or D5LR fluid.
- Obtain blood samples for CBC, chemistries, PT, PTT, coagulation studies, type/Rh, and crossmatch.
- Prepare for possible immediate cesarean delivery.
- Monitor BP, pulse rate and rhythm, respiratory rate, pulse oximetry, fetal heart tones, uterine contractions.

Disposition   Admission to operating suite for cesarean delivery if placenta abruptio is severe. Hospital admission to labor/delivery unit for vaginal delivery may be appropriate with mild placenta abruptio.

Placenta Previa

Etiology
- Abnormally low implanted placenta

Nursing Diagnoses
- Risk for fluid volume deficit

Common Complaints
- Third trimester vaginal bleeding without pain

Triage Rating
- Urgent

Related Factors
- Placenta previa is described according to the degree in which the cervical os is covered by the placenta: partial, marginal, or complete. During effacement and dilation of the cervix in preparation for the delivery process, bleeding from the placenta results.

Assessment Findings
- Possible hypotension
- Possible tachycardia
- Bright red vaginal bleeding
- Normal fetal heart tones

Diagnostics
- Radiographic studies: ultrasound demonstrating a low implanted placenta

Interventions
- Insert IV and infuse NS fluids.
- Obtain blood samples for CBC, type/Rh factor.
- Monitor fetal heart tones, BP, pulse rate and rhythm, respiratory rate, pulse oximetry, continued vaginal bleeding.

Disposition   Hospital admission to labor/delivery unit should be considered for maternal/infant observation.

Pregnancy-Induced Hypertension (PIH)/Eclampsia

Etiology
- Unknown

Nursing Diagnoses
- Altered tissue perfusion: uterine, cerebral
- Risk for injury
- Risk for fluid volume excess

Common Complaints
- Headache, visual disturbances, rapid weight gain, seizure (with eclampsia)

Triage Rating
- Urgent to emergent

Related Factors
- This triad of signs occurs after the twentieth week of pregnancy. The signs that accompany PIH are edema, hypertension, and proteinuria. The hypertension involves an increase in blood pressure of 30 mm Hg systolic and 15 mm Hg diastolic. Placental circulation may become altered and result in fetal compromise. Seizure activity or eclampsia can occur. Associated risk factors include diabetes, multiple pregnancies, substance abuse, and absence of prenatal care. A severe syndrome of PIH is HEELP (hemolysis, elevated liver enzymes, low platelet count) and requires immediate treatment to prevent the development of DIC.

Assessment Findings
- Hypertension
- Edema of hands, feet
- Proteinuria
- Possible increase in deep tendon reflex response
- Possible seizure activity

Diagnostics
- Urinalysis: protein >2+
- Liver enzymes: possible elevation

Interventions
- Place patient in a quiet room and avoid excessive stimulation.
- Insert IV or saline lock.
- Obtain blood samples for CBC, chemistries, PT, PTT, and other studies.
- Consider insertion of indwelling urinary catheter.
- Administer medication to decrease hypertension:
  –**Hydralazine** 20–40 mg IM/IV infusion.
- Administer antiseizure medication:
  –**Magnesium sulfate** 2–4 g IV infusion loading dose.
- Monitor BP, pulse rate and rhythm, respiratory rate, pulse oximetry, deep tendon reflexes, fetal heart tones, urinary output.

Disposition   Patients with mild PIH may be released to home with close follow-up in 24–48 hours with obstetrician. Moderate to severe PIH requires hospital admission to labor/delivery unit for continued monitoring and treatment.

Emergency Childbirth: Uncomplicated*

Etiology
- Impending childbirth

Nursing Diagnoses
- Pain
- Fear

Common Complaints
- Rhythmic uterine contractions, bloody show

Triage Rating
- Urgent to emergent

Related Factors
- The event of childbirth is normal; however, the unprepared environment of the ED may contribute to a stressful delivery. During the actual delivery process, rapid expulsion of the fetus can lead to injury. Therefore the process must be as controlled as possible.

Assessment Findings
- Crowning of the infant's head or bulging at the introitus

Diagnostics
- None

Interventions
- Insert IV or saline lock.
- Obtain blood samples for type/Rh factor test.
- Instruct mother to pant and assist with delivery process.[†]
- Obtain cord blood samples for type/Rh, chemistries.
- Complete documentation and obtain **APGAR**[‡] score at 1 and 5 minutes after delivery.
- Assist with placental delivery.
- Infuse NS or D5LR fluids.
- Massage uterus to stimulate contractions.
- Administer medication to assist with uterine contractions:
  - **Oxytocin** 10 U/1000 mL fluid infusion.
  - **Methylergonovine** 0.2 mg IM.
- Administer **Rho(D) immune globulin** if mother is Rh negative and newborn is Rh positive.
- Monitor BP, pulse rate and rhythm, respiratory rate, pulse oximetry of both mother and newborn, uterine contractions, vaginal bleeding.

*Complications
- Prolapsed cord: elevate mother's hips, administer supplemental oxygen, insert gloved hand into vaginal vault and elevate the head of the fetus away from the cord, transport mother to appropriate area for immediate cesarean delivery.
- Postpartum hemorrhage: if postpartum vaginal bleeding is not controlled with uterine massage, breast feeding, administration of **methylergonovine** or **oxytocin**, transfer patient to operating suite for definitive care.

†Delivery Process
- Extend fingers of dominant hand, placing them on emerging newborn's head. Spread fingers and support the emerging head.
- Apply gentle, firm pressure on emerging head allowing for slow, smooth delivery process.
- As head is delivered, check the neck for presence of umbilical cord. If present, slip cord over head and shoulders. If cord tension is too tight and cannot be slipped over the head, clamp in two places and cut between clamps.
- Suction newborn's airway: nose and mouth.
- As newborn's head spontaneously turns to the side, guide the head downward and deliver anterior shoulder.
- Gently guide the head upward and deliver posterior shoulder.
- Following complete delivery, dry infant and place on or give to mother.
- Clamp umbilical cord in two places and cut between clamps when cord pulsations have stopped.

‡Apgar Score	0	1	2
Heart rate	None	<100	>100
Respiratory rate	None	Irregular	Crying
Muscle tone	Flaccid	Some flexion	Active
Reflexes	None	Weak	Strong
Color	Blue/pale	Blue limbs	Pink

Disposition   Hospital admission to newborn nursery for newly delivered infant. Mother may be observed in ED, then discharged to home or may require hospital admission to postpartum area.

Unit IX

Musculoskeletal Conditions

Acromioclavicular Joint Sprain (Separation)

Etiology
- Fall onto affected shoulder

Nursing Diagnoses
- Pain
- Impaired physical mobility

Common Complaints
- Shoulder pain and limited shoulder motion

Triage Rating
- Nonurgent to urgent

Related Factors
- The degree of sprain or separation is described as first, second, or third. A first degree sprain results in an incomplete tear of the acromioclavicular (AC) ligament without subluxation of the joint. With a second degree sprain, subluxation of the joint is present along with more severe disruption of the surrounding tissues. A third degree sprain involves additional tearing of the coracoclavicular ligaments.

Assessment Findings
- Palpable tenderness over AC joint
- Possible swelling and deformity over injury site
- Limitation of abduction active or passive movement of shoulder

Diagnostics
- Radiographic studies: shoulder film demonstrating minimal to severe upward displacement of the distal clavicle depending on degree of strain

Interventions
- Administer pain relief medications:
  - **Acetaminophen with codeine** PO *or* **hydrocodone** PO *or* **ibuprofen** 600–800 mg PO.
- Place affected upper extremity in arm sling.

Disposition   Release to home and use sling for 1–3 weeks. Instruct patient to remove affected arm from sling a minimun of 3–4 times a day and perform limited shoulder/elbow range of motion exercises. Severe sprains require orthopedic referral for further treatment.

Upper Extremity Bursitis/Tendinitis/Cuff Tear/Tenosynovitis

Etiology
- Inflammation, overuse, trauma

Nursing Diagnoses
- Pain
- Impaired physical mobility
- Risk for infection

Common Complaints
- Pain in affected bursa, swelling over affected bursa, limited movement of shoulder/elbow/wrist

Triage Rating
- Nonurgent

Related Factors
- A bursa is a synovial fluid-filled sac located between muscle, tendon, and bony prominences. There are two types of bursa: superficial and deep. Inflammation can occur from constant friction between the bursa and surrounding structures or infection. Tendinitis can occur before or in association with bursitis. If the tendon sheath is involved, tenosynovitis results. Erythema and warmth of the area indicates a possible infection.

Assessment Findings
- Subacromial bursitis, rotator cuff tear:
  –Limited external rotation; pain at <45 with abduction and internal rotation; positive impingement sign and drop arm test[*]
- Bicipital tendinitis:
  –Palpable tenderness of tendon of long biceps with shoulder externally rotated; reproducible pain with applied resistance when elbow flexed or forearm supinated
- Epicondylitis:
  –Lateral: tenderness, swelling over lateral epicondyle; reproducible pain with wrist extension against resistance
  –Medial: tenderness, swelling over medial epicondyle; reproducible pain with wrist flexion
- Olecranon bursitis:
  –Palpable tenderness over olecranon, swelling
- DeQuervain's tendinitis:
  –Palpable tenderness over radial styloid and possible palpable small nodule; positive Finkelstein's test[†]
- Wrist tendinitis:
  –Palpable linear tenderness over tendon
- Flexor tenosynovitis:
  –Reproducible pain with up lifting of nail of affected digit

Diagnostics
- Radiographic studies: may reveal calcium in bursa; possible high-riding humeral head in rotator cuff tear; soft tissue swelling from inflammation
- Joint aspiration and fluid analysis: if area is warm, erythemic, and swollen, fluid should be analyzed for cell count with differential, gram stain, culture/sensitivity
- CBC: elevation of WBC if infection is present
- Blood culture: consider if infection is present

Interventions
- Administer antiinflammatory medication:
  –**Ibuprofen** 600–800 mg PO.
- Administer antibiotic medication if infection present:
  –**Cefazolin** 1–2 g IM/IV.
  –**Cephalexin** or **dicloxacillin** 500 mg PO.
- Place affected extremity in immobilizer or sling for comfort.

[*]Impingement sign: intermittent pain with flexion and elevation of shoulder (positive with rotator cuff tear); drop arm test: with affected arm abducted to approximately 90 degrees, there is an inability to slowly lower arm to side (positive with rotator cuff tear)

[†]Finkelstein's test: reproducible pain with thumb flexed inside curled fingers and wrist moved toward ulnar side

Disposition   Release to home with instructions of applying ice or heat to affected area and resting affected extremity. Provide referral to an orthopedic surgeon within 3–5 days for further treatment and evaluation. If infection is present, consider hospital admission for continual antibiotic therapy.

Carpal Tunnel Syndrome

Etiology
- Repetitive injury or overuse

Nursing Diagnoses
- Pain

Common Complaints
- Aching pain in first three digits, radial side paresthesia, and numbness; symptoms may be exacerbated at night

Triage Rating
- Nonurgent

Related Factors
- Predisposing factors for developing carpal tunnel syndrome include synovitis of the wrist, repetitive activity of the wrist, pregnancy, and local injury. It is common in adult females >30 years of age.

Assessment Findings
- Possible thenar atrophy in affected hand
- Positive Tinel's sign and Phalen's test*

Diagnostics
- Radiographic studies: wrist films to determine if bony injury is present

Interventions
- Immobilize wrist in splint.
- Administer antiinflammatory medication:
  - **Ibuprofen** 600–800 mg PO.

*Tinel's sign: tapping middle of affected volar wrist produces distal parathesia; Phalen's test: continued flexion of affected wrist for at least 1 minute produces pain and parathesia

Disposition   Release to home with instructions for rest of affected wrist. Provide referral to an orthopedic surgeon or neurologist in 5–7 days.

Acute Sprain

Etiology
• Trauma

Nursing Diagnoses
• Pain
• Impaired physical mobility

Common Complaints
• Pain, swelling surrounding the affected joint, decreased mobility of joint

Triage Rating
• Nonurgent to urgent

Related Factors
• Excessive force applied to a joint can produce stretching or tearing of the ligaments surrounding the joint. Common joint involvement includes the wrist, knee, and ankle. Degree of sprain damage is graded as first (minor tear), second (partial tear), and third (complete tear).

Assessment Findings
• Edema of joint
• Ecchymoses of surrounding soft tissue
• Palpable tenderness over affected ligament
• Possible decreased muscle strength
• Ankle sprain: possible decreased ability to bear weight

Diagnostics
• Radiographic studies:* extremity films demonstrating soft tissue swelling without evidence of fracture

Interventions
• Remove distal constricting jewelry.
• Immobilize and elevate affected extremity.
• Apply ice to affected extremity.
• Administer pain relief medication:
  –**Ibuprofen** 600–800 mg PO *or* **acetaminophen with codeine** PO *or* **hydrocodone** PO.
• Splint affected extremity.
• Provide crutches if lower extremity sprain.
• Monitor swelling, pain relief.

*May use Ottawa Ankle Rules in determining the necessity to obtain radiographic films. Obtain films if any of the following are present:
• Bone tenderness at the posterior edge or tip of lateral malleolus (distal 6 cm) *or*
• Bone tenderness at the posterior edge or tip of the medial malleolus (distal 6 cm) *or*
• Inability to bear weight both immediately after injury or in the ED

Disposition   Release to home with instructions to rest extremity and continue immobilization, ice, and elevation. Third degree sprains require orthopedic consultation, since surgical intervention may be necessary.

Tendon Rupture

Etiology
- Trauma

Nursing Diagnoses
- Pain
- Impaired physical mobility

Common Complaints
- Biceps: sudden sharp pain, bunching of biceps muscle
- Achilles: audible "crack" and pain in heel/calf

Triage Rating
- Urgent

Related Factors
- Lower extremity tendon rupture usually involves the Achilles' tendon. Upper extremity tendon rupture may involve the biceps tendon. In both cases, weakness of the affected muscles will be present.

Assessment Findings
- Biceps:
  - Bunching of biceps muscle
  - Positive Yergason test*
- Achilles:
  - Active plantar flexion may be present
  - Calf squeeze test indicating less motion on ruptured side

Diagnostics
- None

Interventions
- Upper extremity: place extremity in arm sling.
- Lower extremity: place lower leg in posterior mold and provide crutches.
- Administer pain relief medication:
  - **Ibuprofen** 600–800 mg PO.
  - **Acetaminophen with codeine** PO *or* **hydrocodone** PO.

*Yergason test: Patient fully flexes elbow of affected arm. Examiner grasps flexed elbow with one hand and holds wrist with other hand. Patient's arm is externally rotated and a downward pull is applied to the elbow. An unstable biceps tendon will pop out of groove and patient will experience pain.

Disposition   Release to home with follow-up with orthopedic surgeon within 2–3 days for reevaluation.

Fracture

Etiology
- Trauma

Nursing Diagnoses
- Pain
- Impaired physical mobility
- Risk for fluid volume deficit
- Risk for impaired skin integrity
- Altered tissue perfusion

Common Complaints
- Pain, decreased mobility of affected limb, swelling

Triage Rating
- Urgent to emergent

Related Factors
- A fracture occurs when there is a partial or complete disruption of a bone. Fractures may be defined as open (break in the skin) or closed. They are further described according to the anatomic location of the fracture, the direction of the fracture line, angulation of distal bone fragment, and displacement. Blood loss accompanying a fracture may require resuscitation and volume replacement. In children, fractures through either the metaphysis or the epiphysis or both require special care to reduce the possiblity of future growth problems.

Assessment Findings
- Swelling over fracture site and in surrounding soft tissue
- Possible visual deformity of affected bone
- Possible ecchymosis of surrounding tissue
- Palpable tenderness over fracture site

Diagnostics
- Radiographic studies: will demonstrate the majority of fracture sites; comparison views may be required especially in children

Interventions
- Remove distal constricting jewelry.
- Splint affected extremity.
- Apply ice to affected fracture site.
- Elevate affected extremity if possible above the level of the heart.
- Insert IV or saline lock and infuse NS fluid as needed.
- Administer pain relief medication:
  –**Meperidine** 25–100 mg IM/IV *or* **morphine sulfate** 2–10 mg IV *or* **acetaminophen with codeine** PO *or* **hydrocodone** PO.
- Administer antibiotic medication if fracture is open:
  –**Cefazolin** 0.5–2 g IM/IV infusion.
- Administer **dT** 0.5 mL IM as needed.
- Assist with realignment maneuvers as needed.
- Monitor BP, pulse rate and rhythm, respiratory rate, pain relief, neurovascular supply to affected extremity.

Disposition   The majority of patients can be released to home after diagnosis and proper splinting or casting. Patients with lower extremity fractures must be supplied with crutches and given instructions on correct use. Instructions regarding cast care must be emphasized to the patient:
- Keep injured part elevated 12 inches above the heart for the next 48 hours.
- Wiggle toes or fingers of affected extremity at least once per hour.
- If excessive blueness, paleness, or coolness of extremity occurs, return to ED immediately.
- Keep follow-up appointment with physician.

Hospital admission is required for fractures in which complications such as compartmental syndrome, bone necrosis or fat emboli are common. Unstable fractures such as Salter III, IV, and V or grossly displaced fractures require surgical intervention. Patients with open fractures and intraarticular fractures require close follow-up with an orthopedic surgeon within 24 hours if hospital admission is not viable.

Common Fractures

Affected Bone	Assessment Findings	Suggested Treatment
• Clavicle	• Shoulder drops inward, downward, or forward	• Arm sling
• Proximal humerus	• Loss of internal rotation/abduction	• Nondisplaced: shoulder immobilizer
		• Displaced or accompanying dislocation: immediate consulation
• Elbow	• Posterior fat pad on x-ray examination	• Distal humerus: splint with arm at 45-degree angle/supination
		• Olecranon process: surgery within 6–8 hours
		• Olecranon process and dislocation: immediate consultation
• Radius/ulna	• Painful pronation-supination movement	• Nondisplaced: volar splint and sling
	• Monteggia's: fracture of ulna and radial head dislocation	• Immediate consultation
	• Galeazzi's: radial head fracture and disruption of distal radioulnar joint	• Immediate consultation
	• Colles': distal radius with dorsal displacement and shortening	• Orthopedic consultation
	• Smith's: distal radius with volar displacement and shortening	• Orthopedic consultation
• Carpal-metacarpal	• Scaphoid: tenderness over anatomical "snuff box"	• Thumb spica splint
	• Bennett's: fracture of distal thumb and dislocation of thumb carpometacarpal joint	• Orthopedic consultation
	• Metacarpal shaft	• Ulnar gutter splint for fracture of 4 or 5 metacarpals
		• Volar splint for other metacarpal fracture
	• Metacarpal neck (Boxer's): involve fourth and fifth metacarpals and are often open	• Closed: volar splint
		• Open: orthopedic consultation
• Thumb/finger	• Tenderness over fracture site	• Proximal fracture: splint finger in extension. Distal fracture: splint finger in position of function
	• PIP joint and >25% of articular surface involved or V shape	• Orthopedic consultation
• Pelvis	• Hypovolemia symptoms from volume loss; iliac mobility	• Hemodynamic stabilization; orthopedic consultation
• Hip	• Affected leg externally rotated and shortened	• Orthopedic consultation
• Femur	• Affected leg shortened, severe muscle spasm	• Application of traction splint; orthopedic consultation
• Patella	• Effusion, inability to extend knee; sunrise x-ray view is helpful	• Nondisplaced: aspiration of effusion, knee immobilizer, crutches
		• Displaced: orthopedic consultation
• Proximal or mid tibia/fibula	• Usually fractured together and can develop into compartmental syndrome	• Orthopedic consultation
• Ankle	• Pain with extension, flexion, and weight bearing; may be single malleolar, bimalleolar, or trimalleolar fracture	• Nondisplaced: posterior mold and crutches
		• Displaced: orthopedic consultation
	• Dupuytren's fracture: fibula fracture 7–10 cm above ankle	
	• Maisonneuve fracture: proximal fibular neck	
• Tarsometatarsal	• Instability of forefoot	• Immediate orthopedic consultation
• Metatarsal	• With stress fracture, x-ray examination may appear normal	• Nondisplaced: posterior mold, crutches
		• Displaced: orthopedic consultation
• Calcaneus	• Heel may appear widened with a decreased height; possible associated T-12, L-1, L-2 compression fractures	• Orthopedic consultation
• Toe	• Edema, ecchymosis, tenderness over fracture site	• Nondisplaced great toe: U splint with plantar slab and crutches
		• Displaced great toe: orthopedic consultation
		• Lesser toes: buddy tape, hard sole shoe

Joint Dislocation/Subluxation

Etiology
- Trauma

Nursing Diagnoses
- Pain
- Altered tissue perfusion

Common Complaints
- Pain in affected joint; decreased mobility of joint; "popping," "snapping," or "tearing" sounds heard at time of injury

Triage Rating
- Urgent to emergent

Related Factors
- A joint disruption with loss of contact between the articulating surfaces is termed a dislocation or luxation. When only partial loss of contact occurs, the injury is termed a subluxation. Large joint dislocations have the potential to impinge on surrounding nerves and vascular structures. Relocation of the joint is the goal of treatment.

Assessment Findings
- Noticeable deformity of involved joint
- Palpable tenderness of affected joint
- Decreased mobility of affected joint
- Positive apprehension tests especially of knee or shoulder*
- Possible edema and ecchymoses of surrounding soft tissues
- Normal or diminished neurovascular supply to distal tissues

Diagnostics
- Radiographic studies: will demonstrate joint dislocation; subluxation may not be evident on film†

Interventions
- Remove distal constricting jewelry.
- Splint joint and extremity in position "as it lays" if neurovascular supply is intact.
- Consider insertion of IV or saline lock if dislocation of large joint.
- Administer medication to relieve pain:
  - **Midazolam** 2–5 mg IV.
  - **Diazepam** 5–10 mg IV.
- Assist with relocation of joint.
- Immobilize joint.
- Monitor BP, pulse rate and rhythm, respiratory rate, pulse oximetry, pain relief, distal neurovascular supply.

*Apprehension test: assists in identifying chronic dislocation
- Shoulder: abduct and externally rotate arm to position where shoulder is ready to dislocate; a noticeable look of apprehension or alarm on patient's face along with resistance of further motion is a positive test
- Patella: with patient supine, legs flat, and quadriceps relaxed, press against medial border of patella. If patella begins to dislocate, apprehension and distress will be evident in patient's face

†Subluxation of the radial head (nursemaid's elbow) is a common condition in children ages 1–4 years. The typical history involves a sudden pulling on the child's arm resulting in the child not moving the affected arm. Pain is present. Radiographic studies are not required. Relocation is easily attempted by the examiner placing his/her fingers on the posterior radial head while also anchoring his/her thumb in the antecubital fossa of the affected arm. In one coordinated motion, supinate the forearm, quickly flex the elbow, and move the flexed forearm toward the shoulder of the affected arm. A palpable "pop" signaling relocation should be felt.

Disposition   If relocation is successful, release patient to home with close follow-up in 2–3 days by primary care physician or orthopedic surgeon. If relocation is not successful, immediate consultation with an orthopedic surgeon is necessary.

Lower Back Pain

Etiology
- Trauma, infection, systemic disease

Nursing Diagnoses
- Pain
- Impaired physical mobility

Common Complaints
- Pain, muscle spasms, decreased mobility

Triage Rating
- Nonurgent to urgent

Related Factors
- Back pain may be a result of direct injury to the spinal column or progressive disk disease. Other considerations, especially in the older population, are systemic conditions such as metastatic disease and abdominal aneurysm. Psychological conditions must also be considered as a cause for chronic back pain. If neurologic function loss or impairment is present, such as incontinence, presence of saddle anesthesia, decreased deep tendon reflexes, diminished or unequal sensation or motor movement, or true radiculopathy, a more serious problem exists.

Assessment Findings
- Possible asymmetrical gait
- Restricted mobility of the lower back
- Positive radiculopathy:
  –Passive flexion of hip produces radicular pain in leg
  –Crossed leg raise produces radicular pain in leg not raised
- Possible tenderness and tenseness of paravertebral muscles

Diagnostics
- Radiographic studies: consider if patient is >50 years, radiculopathy or neurologic findings are present, or there is a history of metastatic disease, bony vertebral tenderness, or use of steroids; CT scan if abdominal aneurysm is possible

Interventions
- Administer pain relief medications:
  –**Ketorolac** 30–60 mg IM *or* **meperidine** 50–100 mg IM *or* **morphine sulfate** 5–10 mg IM.
- Monitor BP, pulse rate and rhythm, respiratory rate, pulse oximetry, pain relief, mobility improvement.

Disposition   The majority of patients with lower back pain are released to home with prescriptions for continued pain relief and follow-up in 3–5 days. The patient should be instructed to use cold therapy for 20–30 minutes several times a day for the first 24 hours and then begin heat therapy. Strict bed rest is no longer encouraged unless it is for a short time to treat acute pain. If systemic disease is the cause of back pain or if pain relief is not achieved with ED treatment, hospital admission should be considered.

Septic Arthritis

Etiology
- Bacterial, viral organisms

Nursing Diagnoses
- Pain
- Infection
- Impaired physical mobility

Common Complaints
- Pain, swelling, redness, tenderness of affected joint

Triage Rating
- Urgent

Related Factors
- A common pathogen that causes a septic joint is the gonococcal organism. There may be no associated genital discharge. Whatever the offending organism, the condition is usually monoarthritic and affects the large joints. Aspiration of fluid from the joint and subsequent tests will assist in identifying the primary cause of the infection.

Assessment Findings
- Possible increased temperature
- Possible tachycardia
- Affected joint:
  - Edema
  - Erythema
  - Tenderness
  - Warmth to touch

Diagnostics
- Radiographic studies: will assist in determining coexisting injury
- Joint fluid aspiration: cell count elevation if bacterial organism; gram stain may assist in identifying organism; culture and sensitivity will not be immediately available; crystals may be present if gout is the cause
- CBC: elevated WBC if bacterial cause
- Sedimentation rate: may be elevated
- Blood cultures: results not available during ED treatment

Interventions
- Insert IV or saline lock.
- Obtain blood samples for CBC, sedimentation rate, culture.
- Assist with joint fluid aspiration.
- Administer antibiotic medication as needed:
  - **Cefazolin** 1–2 g IV/IM.
  - **Penicillin G** 2–4 million units IV infusion.
- Monitor BP, pulse rate and rhythm, respiratory rate, pulse oximetry.

Disposition   Consider hospital admission if patient is febrile. Patients with minor viral organism, gout inflammation, and no surrounding cellulitis may be released to home with close follow-up within 24 hours.

Compartmental Syndrome

Etiology
- Circular plaster casts, snake bite, circumferential burns, soft tissue injury, fracture

Nursing Diagnoses
- Pain
- Altered tissue perfusion

Common Complaints
- Increasing pain in affected extremity, decreased mobility of affected extremity

Triage Rating
- Urgent to emergent

Related Factors
- The anatomic compartments most frequently affected by this syndrome are in the lower leg, forearm, and interosseous space of the hands. When pressure inside a limited compartment space is increased from internal swelling or prolonged external pressure, circulation to tissues within the compartmental space decreases. Normal compartment pressure measures <20 mm Hg. Pressures >40 mm Hg require immediate surgical decompression.

Assessment Findings
- Pain in affected extremity especially with passive movement
- Diminished pulse in affected extremity
- Increased pallor of affected extremity
- Decreased sensation in affected extremity

Diagnostics
- Radiologic studies: may demonstrate reason for compartmental syndrome such as proximal tibia/fibula fracture
- Pressure measurement of compartment: readings >30 mm Hg

Interventions
- Elevate affected extremity only to level of patient's heart.
- Insert IV or saline lock.
- Remove any constricting dressings or casts.
- Administer pain relief medication: **–Meperidine** 25–100 mg IV/IM.
- Assist with measurement of compartmental pressure.
- Monitor BP, pulse rate and rhythm, respiratory rate, pulse oximetry, pain relief, neurovascular changes of affected extremity.

Disposition   Hospital admission is required for either immediate surgical decompression or continued monitoring of the neurovascular supply to the affected extremity.

Crush Injury

Etiology
- Trauma

Nursing Diagnoses
- Pain
- Altered tissue perfusion

Common Complaints
- Pain, swelling of injured area

Triage Rating
- Urgent to emergent

Related Factors
- This type of injury results in muscle and tissue damage. Vascular and nerve structures may also be damaged. Complications include tubular necrosis, infection, hemorrhage, and compartmental syndrome.

Assessment Findings
- Ecchymosis and hematoma formation surrounding injured area
- Possible deformity if extremity involvement

Diagnostics
- Urinalysis: presence of myoglobin if rhabdomyolysis is present
- Radiographic studies: injured extremity for possible fracture

Interventions
- Apply pressure dressing to crushed area for control of blood loss.
- If extremity involved, elevate area.
- Gently cleanse area with NS.
- Insert IV and infuse NS fluid to maintain urinary output at 100–300 mL/h.
- Administer **dT** 0.5 mL IM as needed.
- Monitor BP, pulse rate and rhythm, respiratory rate, pulse oximetry, urinary output.

Disposition   If minor crush injury to extremity is present without coexisting fracture, release to home. If moderate to severe crush injury or fracture is present, hospital admission to medical/surgical area is required.

Amputation

Etiology
- Trauma

Nursing Diagnoses
- Pain
- Altered tissue perfusion
- Impaired skin integrity
- Risk for fluid volume deficit

Common Complaints
- Pain, obvious injury

Triage Rating
- Urgent to emergent

Related Factors
- Any life-threatening condition co-existing with an amputated body part must be attended to first. After life-threatening conditions have been stabilized, attention can be directed toward preservation of the amputated part and stump care. Amputations commonly involve extremities or digits and are associated with crush injury or industrial and farm accidents. The amputation may be partial or complete, with fluid loss being more significant with a partial amputation. If an amputation occurs to the hand or fingers, determine if the involved part is the patient's dominant hand.

Assessment Findings
- Active bleeding from injury site
- Obvious partial or complete amputation

Diagnostics
- Radiographic studies: film of the partial amputated body part or stump possibly demonstrating the presence of foreign objects or fracture

Interventions
- Insert IV and infuse NS fluid if fluid deficit is present.
- Obtain blood samples as needed.
- Administer pain relief medication:
  –**Bupivacaine** or **lidocaine (Xylocaine)** digital block or both if appropriate.
  –**Meperidine** 25–100 mg IM/IV.
- Administer antibiotic medication:
  –**Cefazolin** 0.5–2 g IM/IV.
- Administer **dT** 0.5 mL IM as required.
- Stump care:
  –Control active bleeding without the use of tourniquets or clamps.
  –Rinse stump with NS solution.
  –Cover area with saline-moistened sponges and bulky sterile dressing.
  –Splint and elevate extremity.
- Amputated part care:
  –Collect all amputated parts if possible.
  –Minimally rinse part(s) to remove gross contamination.
  –Wrap part(s) in sterile gauze (dry or minimally moistened with NS solution). Do not soak parts.
  –Place wrapped parts in a sealable plastic bag.
  –Place plastic bag on ice.
  –Label bag with patient identification.
- Assist with repair of stump.
- Monitor BP, pulse rate and rhythm, respiratory rate, pulse oximetry, continued bleeding, pain relief.

Disposition   Depending on the location of the amputation and other injuries, the patient may be released to home or transferred to a replantation center. If the patient is released to home, instructions regarding wound care and close follow-up must be addressed.

Unit X

Skin Injury/Rash Conditions

Minor Skin Injury

Laceration
- Tear in the skin over a bony prominence. Extent and type of laceration varies in length and depth. Repair is usually by primary closure.

Incision
- Cut in the skin made by an object. Extent and depth of incision varies. Repair is usually by primary closure.

Abrasion
- Denudation of skin extending through partial-thickness skin layers. Healing is through secondary intention.

Avulsion
- Full-thickness tissue loss. Healing is through secondary intention and may require skin grafting.

Contusion
- Collection of blood under tissue without break in skin integrity.

Interventions
- Any injury that results in a break in skin integrity requires thorough irrigation and cleaning prior to any repair procedures.
- Anesthetizing the wound may be necessary before cleansing. This may be obtained with local infiltration, topical anesthesia, or digital or regional anesthesia.
- Lacerations and incisions may require suturing.*
- Address the need for tetanus immunization[†] and antibiotic medication.
- Apply sterile dressings in three layers (contact layer with nonadhering material, intermediate layer with absorbable material, and outer layer for protection) to assist in protecting the wound.
- Give all patients wound care instruction sheets.

*Suturing Guidelines

Location	Material	Removal
Scalp	3–0, 4–0 nylon	7–12 days
Ear pinna	6–0 nylon, 5–0 Vicryl in perichondrium	4–6 days
Eyelid	6–0 nylon	3–5 days
Lip	4–0 silk (mucosa), 6–0 nylon (skin), 5–0 Vicryl (SC, muscle)	3–5 days
Face	6–0 nylon (skin), 4 or 5–0 Vicryl (SC)	3–5 days
Neck	5–0 nylon (skin), 4–0 Vicryl (SC)	4–6 days
Trunk	4 or 5–0 nylon (skin), 4–0 Vicryl (SC, fat)	7–12 days
Extremity	4 or 5–0 nylon (skin), 3 or 4–0 Vicryl (SC, fat, muscle)	7–14 days
Hands/feet	4 or 5–0 nylon	7–12 days

†Tetanus Prophylaxis in Wound Management

Clean Wound
- **dT: No** only if known 3 or more previous doses and less than 10 years since last dose. Otherwise, **Yes**.
- **TIG: No**

All Other Wounds
- **dT: No** only if known 3 or more previous doses and less than 5 years since last dose. Otherwise, **Yes**.
- **TIG: No** if same criteria as above; otherwise, **Yes**.

Subungual Hematoma

Etiology
- Trauma

Common Complaints
- Pain, throbbing of affected finger

Related Factors
- A hematoma under the nail bed usually results from blunt injury to the finger.

Nursing Diagnoses
- Pain

Triage Rating
- Nonurgent

Assessment Findings
- Nail bed hematoma
- Palpable tenderness of affected nail

Diagnostics
- Radiographic studies: digit film will determine if a coexisting fracture is present

Interventions
- Use an 18-gauge needle, heated paper clip, or disposable cautery and make a hole in the nail over the hematoma. Blood will be released with immediate pain relief.

Disposition   Release to home with wound care instructions.

Abscess

Etiology
- Bacterial organism

Nursing Diagnoses
- Pain
- Infection

Common Complaints
- Pain in abscess area, surrounding warmth, fever

Triage Rating
- Nonurgent

Related Factors
- The most common offending organism involved in a cutaneous abcess is *Staphylococcus aureus*. Bacteria may enter the skin through a hair follicle, break in the skin integrity through injury, or subcutaneous ("skin popping") drug use. The result is a localized collection of pus. Surrounding cellulitis may be present. The condition of *hidradenitis suppurativa* is a carbuncle (widely spread lesion with suppuration and pus draining ports). It is commonly located in the axilla or groin and involves sweat glands. This condition does not require incision and drainage, only antibiotic therapy.

Assessment Findings
- Tender cutaneous mass with erythema and possible fluctuance
- Possible surrounding cellulitis or lymphangitic streaking
- Possible increased temperature
- Tachycardia

Diagnostics
- Possible gram stain and culture and sensitivity of removed pus
- CBC: possible elevated WBC from infection

Interventions
- Insert IV or saline lock if large abscess or surrounding cellulitis or lymphangitic streaking is present.
- Administer medication prior to incision and drainage:
  –Possible conscious sedation with **midazolam** 2–5 mg IV.
  –**Fentanyl** 2–3 µg/kg up to 50 µg/kg IV *or* **ketamine** 1–2 mg/kg IV or 4 mg/kg IM.
  –Pain relief with **meperidine** 25–100 mg IV/IM.
- Assist with incision and drainage procedure followed by irrigation and packing.
- Administer antibiotic medication as needed:
  –**Cefazolin** 0.5–2 g IM/IV infusion.
  –**Dicloxacillin** 500 mg PO.
- Monitor BP, pulse rate and rhythm, respiratory rate, pulse oximetry, pain relief.

Disposition   The majority of patients can be released to home with instructions for follow-up in 1–2 days for recheck and repacking of abscess. If extensive cellulitis is present, consider hospital admission for continual antibiotic therapy.

Cellulitis

Etiology
- Bacterial organism

Nursing Diagnoses
- Infection

Common Complaints
- Fever, cutaneous area of redness and warmth

Triage Rating
- Urgent

Related Factors
- The most common bacterial organisms causing this diffuse cutaneous and subcutaneous inflammation are *Staphylococcus aureus* and *Haemophilus influenzae*. Frequently, a preceding wound allows an entrance site for the bacteria.

Assessment Findings
- Possible increased temperature
- Diffuse area on skin of erythema, warmth
- Possible enlarged proximal lymphadenopathy and "streaking"

Diagnostics
- CBC: elevated WBC indicating infection
- Blood culture: results will not be available for ED treatment
- If over joint space: aspiration of joint fluid for cell count with differential, gram stain, culture/sensitivity

Interventions
- Insert IV or saline lock if IV antibiotic medications are required.
- Administer antibiotic medications:
  - **Cefazolin** 0.5–2 g IM/IV infusion.
  - **Cephalexin** 500 mg PO (Peds: 75–100 mg/kg/d).
  - **Dicloxacillin** 500 mg PO (Peds: 12–25 mg/kg/d).

Disposition
The majority of patients can be released to home with close follow-up in 24 hours. Patients who require admission for continued antibiotic therapy include those with:
- Extensive cellulitis or systemic toxicity
- Diminished arterial pulse in an extremity
- Cutaneous necrosis
- Closed space infections of the hand
- Periorbital cellulitis
- Immunosuppression or diabetes

Impetigo

Etiology
- Bacterial organism

Nursing Diagnoses
- Infection
- Impaired skin integrity

Common Complaints
- Weeping rash

Triage Rating
- Nonurgent

Related Factors
- Begins as small superficial vesicles with a fragile roof. The roof is quickly lost, allowing the vesicles to rupture, leaving the typical "honey-colored" crust. The common bacteria involved is *Staphylococcus* or *Streptococcus aureus*. The most common sites include the face and extremities but may occur in any location. Children are affected more frequently than adults.

Assessment Findings
- Solitary or multiple red papules and weepy vesicles with "honey-colored" crust

Diagnostics
- None

Interventions
- Administer antibiotic medication:
  –**Dicloxacillin** 250–500 mg PO (Peds: 12–25 mg/kg/d).

Disposition Release to home with follow-up in 1 week.

Scarlatina

Etiology
- Bacterial organism

Nursing Diagnoses
- Infection

Common Complaints
- Fever, sore throat, rash, headache

Triage Rating
- Urgent

Related Factors
- The rash of scarlatina is a vascular response to the circulating exotoxin from group A hemolytic *Streptococcus* and to a lesser extent *Staphylococcus*. The incubation period is 3–5 days, and the patient is not considered infectious within 24 hours after the onset of antibiotic therapy. Complications include otitis media, glomerulonephritis, rheumatic fever, sinusitis, and bacteremia.

Assessment Findings
- Increased temperature
- Rash:
  - Pinhead size lesions on an erythematous base that blanch
  - Palpable texture of sandpaper
  - Generalized pattern but absent from face
  - Linear petechiae in skin folds of axilla and antecubital space
- Thick, white coating on tongue (strawberry tongue)
- Generalized lymphadenopathy

Diagnostics
- Possible throat culture

Interventions
- Administer antibiotic medication:
  - **Penicillin V** 500 mg PO (Peds: 40–60 mg/kg/d) *or* **benzathine penicillin G**:
    - *Adults*: 1.2 million units IM
    - *<60 pounds*: 600,000 units IM
    - *60–90 pounds*: 900,000 units IM.
  - **Dicloxacillin** 15–20 mg/kg/d PO if staphylococcal.*

*Differentiation of staphylococcal rash:
- No strawberry tongue
- Skin often painful or tender

Disposition   Release to home with follow-up in 7–10 days.

Viral Rashes

Herpes Simplex
- Age group: children, adolescents, adults
- Onset: tingling, stinging prodrome for few hours to 1–2 days prior to appearance of lesions
- Appearance: vesicular clusters on mucous membranes or face
- Duration: self-limited, 2 or more weeks
- Treatment: **acyclovir** 200 mg, 2 tablets tid × 7 days

Herpes Zoster
- Age group: usually adults >50 years of age
- Onset: acute prodromal pains, followed by skin lesions
- Appearance: unilateral grouped vesicles following dermatome pattern
- Duration: 3 weeks
- Treatment: **acyclovir** 800 mg, 5 times a day × 7 days

Varicella
- Age group: all ages, but common in childhood
- Onset: viral prodrome with fever, myalgia, chills, arthralgias 3 days prior
- Appearance: single, small lesions in progressing stages of papules, vesicles, pustules, crusting. Crops erupt for 4–5 days and are crusted by 1 week. Usually starts on trunk and spreads to face and extremities
- Duration: 1–3 weeks
- Treatment: severe or complicating disease: **acyclovir** 800 mg, 5 times a day × 7 days (Peds: 20 mg/kg/d). Otherwise symptomatic treatment with **acetaminophen, diphenhydramine.** Administration of **varicella-zoster immune globulin (VZIG)** within 72–96 hours after exposure may prevent or diminish the disease

Hand-Foot-and-Mouth Disease
- Age group: infants and children
- Onset: acute with oral lesions
- Appearance: widespread or grouped red-ringed vesicles. Quickly progressing to painful erosions on intraoral mucosa, tongue, hard palate. Lesions are also found on fingers, toes, hands, and feet including soles, and palms
- Duration: self-limited, 7–10 days
- Treatment: symptomatic with analgesics, **acetaminophen,** topical **lidocaine (Xylocaine Viscous),** and swish and swallow **diphenhydramine elixir**

Viral Exanthem
- Age group: children
- Onset: prodrome of rhinorrhea, fever
- Appearance: differing patterns, but frequently generalized maculopapular lesions
- Duration: varies
- Treatment: symptomatic with **acetaminophen**

Rubeola
- Age group: children, adolescents
- Onset: 1- to 4-day prodrome of cough, coryza, conjunctivitis (3 Cs), fever
- Appearance: deep red macular rash beginning on face and neck, then spreading to trunk and extremities. Small, bluish white spots on buccal mucosa (Koplik's spots)
- Duration: 3–4 days
- Treatment: vitamin A, symptomatic with **acetaminophen**

Rubella
- Age group: any unvaccinated age group
- Onset: prodrome 1–3 days of enlarged cervical, posterior, and postauricular lymph nodes; fever; sore throat; headache; malaise
- Appearance: pink, maculopapular rash beginning on face, then spreading to trunk and extremities
- Duration: 3–4 days
- Treatment: symptomatic with **acetaminophen**

Roseola
- Age group: children <3 years of age
- Onset: 3- to 4-day prodrome of fever
- Appearance: pink maculopapular rash beginning on trunk and spreading to face and extremities
- Duration: 1–2 days
- Treatment: symptomatic with **acetaminophen**

Candidiasis

- Age group: all ages
- Appearance:
  –Oral cavity: white plaque on erythematous base on tongue, trachea, esophagus
  –Diaper area: beefy red, well-demarcated lesions with well-defined margins and satellite lesions
  –Body folds: often seen in obese individuals; occurs in skinfolds of axilla, abdomen, under the breasts, inguinal area; red, moist, plaque or papules
  –Vagina: thick, white, cheesy discharge
  –Penis: more common in uncircumcised males; multiple, round red erosion lesions on glans and shaft
  –Nails: often result of thumb sucking; erythema and swelling at nail base
- Treatment: **nystatin**
  –Oral: oral suspension 2–6 mL qid × 7–10 days
  –Diaper: cream 3-4 times per day × 7–10 days
  –Body folds: cream 3–4 times per day × 7–10 days
  –Vagina: vaginal suppositories or cream × 7 days
  –Penis: cream 2–3 times per day × 10 days
  –Nails: cream nightly × 3–4 weeks

Tinea

- Versicolor: most common in adolescence and young adults
  –Appearance: multiple, small, circular macules of differing colors; most common on trunk
  –Treatment: **selenium sulfide** 2.5% lotion applied at night and removed in morning *or* **clotrimazole** 1% cream bid × 4 weeks
- Capitis: most common in prepubertal children
  –Appearance: erythema and scaling of scalp, patchy hair loss; kerion (tender, boggy, lesion) may be present
  –Treatment: **selenium sulfide** 2.5% shampoo 2 times per week × 2 weeks
- Corporis: all age groups
  –Appearance: circular, erythematous, well-demarcated lesions with a raised, scaly, vesicular border; central area is paler in color
  –Treatment: **clotrimazole** 1% cream bid × 2 weeks
- Pedis: common in adolescents and adults
  –Appearance: vesiculopustular, fine, scaly lesions between the toes
  –Treatment: **clotrimazole** 1% cream bid × 2 weeks

Hypersensitivity Rashes

Etiology
- Allergy, immune response

Nursing Diagnoses
- Risk for impaired skin integrity

Common Complaints
- Acute rash, possible itching

Triage Rating
- Nonurgent to urgent

Related Factors
- The most common diagnoses associated with hypersensitivity reactions are urticaria, erythema multiforme, and erythema nodosum. Urticaria is associated with allergy; erythema multiforme with medications, infection, pregnancy, connective tissue disease, and malignancies; erythema nodosum with tuberculosis and streptococcal infections in children, and sarcoidosis in adults.

Assessment Findings
- Urticaria:
  - Localized raised lesions with well-demarcated borders
  - Pruritus
  - Possible angioedema
- Erythema multiforme:
  - Target lesions and papules
  - Dusky red, round symmetric maculopapule lesions on back of hands and feet and extensor aspect of forearms and legs
- Erythema nodosum:
  - Red, nodelike swelling over shins
  - Lesion border poorly defined
  - Lesions painful, hard

Diagnostics
- Sedimentation rate: elevated with erythema nodosum
- Radiographic studies: consider chest films in patients with erythema nodosum

Interventions
- Administer medication to diminish symptoms:
  - Urticaria:
    - **Epinephrine** 0.3–0.5 mL 1:1000 solution SC (Peds: 0.01 mg/kg).
    - **Diphenhydramine** 25–100 mg IM/IV/PO (Peds: 5 mg/kg/d).
    - **Hydroxyzine** 0.5 mg/kg up to 25–50 mg IM/PO.
    - **Cimetidine** 300 mg IV/IM/PO.
  - Erythema multiforme:
    - **Prednisone** 40–80 mg/d PO.
  - Erythema nodosum:
    - **Indomethacin** 25–50 mg PO *or* **naproxen** 200–500 mg PO.

Disposition
Release to home.

Infestation Rashes

Scabies

- Age group: all ages
- Appearance: common areas are hand, wrists, groin, axillae, waist. Red papulovesicles in short-track lines. Secondary infection is common.
- Treatment: **pemethrin cream** applied to total body below the head, then removed in 8–14 hours. Household members should be treated prophylactically.

Pediculosis (Lice)

- Age group: all ages, but most common in school-aged children
- Appearance: most common in hair near nape of neck. White nits at base of hair shafts. Pubic lice appear crablike.
- Treatment: **pemethrin 1% cream** applied to shampooed and towel dried hair and left for 10 minutes, then rinsed. Use fine-tooth comb to assist in removal of nits. Household contacts should also be treated.

Nail Infections

Paronychia

- Inflammation and collection of pus inside the fingernail fold. Usual cause is *Staphylococcus aureus*.

- Treatment: anesthetize area with ethyl chloride or digital block. Elevate affected nail cuticle where infection exists with a #11 scalpel blade. Drain pus. Antibiotic therapy not required.

Ingrown Toenail

- Acute or chronic inflammation of toenail margin caused by the nail growing into overhanging skin. The usual cause is incorrect cutting of toenails, either too aggressively or in convex shape.

- Treatment: anesthetize toe using a digital block. Cut toenail away from irritated skin and remove nail spur out from under the overhanging skin. Antibiotics are not required.

Lyme Disease

Etiology
- Spirochete

Nursing Diagnoses
- Impaired skin integrity
- Infection

Common Complaints
- Rash, weakness, "flulike" symptoms

Triage Rating
- Nonurgent

Related Factors
- *Borrelia burgdorferi* is the spirochete responsible for Lyme disease. It is transmitted by the *Ixodes dammini* tick, which is carried by small mammals and deer. The highest incidence in the United States is in the northeast, north midwest, and western states. The characteristic rash is not always present, and the late-stage symptoms may not appear until months or years after the tick bite, although the usual incubation period is 3–32 days.

Assessment Findings
- Possible characteristic rash: reddened rash with "bull's-eye" center
- Bradycardia with possible heart block
- Possible Bell's palsy
- Possible neck meningism

Diagnostics
- ELISA or Western blot test: may give false-positive results
- ECG: may demonstrate cardiac dysrhythmia

Interventions
- Remove tick if still present.
- Mild case:
  –Administer antibiotic medication:
  - **Doxycycline** 100 mg PO (not recommended for children) *or* **tetracycline** 500 mg PO (not recommended for children).
  - **Amoxicillin** 25–50 mg/kg for children.
- Severe case:
  –Insert IV or saline lock.
  –Administer antibiotic medication:
  - **Ceftriaxone** 0.5–2 g IV infusion.
  - **Penicillin G** high dose IV infusion.
- Monitor BP, pulse rate and rhythm.

Disposition   Patients with a mild case can be released to home with instructions about preventing future tick bites. Patients with severe cases require hospital admission for continued antibiotic therapy and cardiac monitoring.

Rocky Mountain Spotted Fever

Etiology
- *Rickettsia* organism

Nursing Diagnoses
- Impaired skin integrity
- Infection

Common Complaints
- Fever, joint pain, rash, headache

Triage Rating
- Urgent to emergent

Related Factors
- The infecting agent is *Rickettsia rickettsii*. The highest incidence in the United States is encountered in the south Atlantic, south central states, and Oklahoma. The incubation period is approximately 1 week. If untreated shock and death can occur if treatment is delayed 6 or more days.

Assessment Findings
- Increased temperature
- Conjunctival irritation
- Maculopapular rash starts on extremities (hand palms and feet soles) then spreads to trunk, neck, and face
- Petechial rash may be present in 4 days

Diagnostics
- CBC: usually normal
- Chemistries: hyponatremia, hypochloremia, and hypoalbuminemia may be present
- Possible lumbar puncture: CSF usually normal

Interventions
- Mild case:
  –Obtain blood samples for CBC, chemistries as needed.
  –Administer antibiotic medication:
  - **Doxycycline** 200 mg PO loading dose *or* **tetracycline** 25–50 mg/kg PO *or* **chloramphenicol** 50–100 mg/kg PO.
- Severe case:
  –Insert IV and infuse NS fluid.
  –Obtain blood samples for CBC, chemistries, blood coagulopathies.
  –Assist with lumbar puncture as indicated.
  –Administer antibiotic medication:
  - **Chloramphenicol** 50–100 mg/kg IV infusion.
- Monitor BP, pulse rate and rhythm, respiratory rate, pulse oximetry, urinary output.

Disposition   Hospital admission should be considered for all patients, even those with a mild case.

Mammalian Bites

Etiology
- Humans, dogs, cats

Nursing Diagnoses
- Pain
- Impaired skin integrity
- Risk for infection

Common Complaints
- Pain, open puncture wound, redness surrounding wound

Triage Rating
- Nonurgent to urgent

Related Factors
- Transmission of bacteria from the mouth of a human, dog, or cat into a wound can lead to infection. *Pasteurella multocida* is the infectious agent in 20–50% of dog bites and 80% of cat bites. In addition, rabies may also be transmitted to humans through dog bites. Human bites can transmit hepatitis B, *Staphylococcus,* and *Streptococcus* organisms. Bites inflicted by children carry a lower risk of infection because of a lower bacteria count in the mouth.

Assessment Findings
- Obvious puncture wound injury with possible tearing of surrounding tissues

Diagnostics
- None

Interventions
- Control bleeding from wound with direct pressure.
- Thoroughly irrigate wound.
- Assist with suture repair only if low-risk bite or for cosmetic reasons.
- Administer antibiotic medication as required:
  - Dog bite:
    - **Penicillin V** 500 mg PO (Peds: 25–50 mg/kg/d) *or* **dicloxacillin** 500 mg PO (Peds: 12–25 mg/kg/d) *or* **amoxicillin-clavulanate** 500 mg PO (Peds: 40 mg/kg/d).
  - Cat bite:
    - **Amoxicillin-clavulanate** 500 mg PO (Peds: 40 mg/kg/d).
  - Human bite:
    - **Penicillin V** 500 mg PO (Peds: 25–50 mg/kg/d).
- Administer **dT** 0.5 mL IM if necessary.
- If suspicion of rabies consider:
  - **Human diploid cell vaccine** 1 mL IM and repeated on days 3, 7, 14, 28 *and* **rabies immune globulin** 20 IU/kg with $1/2$ infiltrated into wound and $1/2$ IM.
- Report incident to proper authorities.

Disposition   Release to home with close follow-up in 24 hours unless infection necessitates hospital admission. Provide instructions regarding wound care at home.

Spider Bites

Black Widow

- Injects neurotoxic venom
- Swelling at venom injection site
- Pain at site within 15–60 minutes, then progressing to chest pain, back and shoulder pain, *or* abdominal pain with rigidity
- Treatment usually symptomatic for pain relief, although antivenin may be necessary. Administration of 10% calcium gluconate, diazepam, or methocarbamol is controversial as to effectiveness for control of muscle spasm and pain.

Brown Recluse

- Injects cytotoxic venom
- Sharp pain at instant of bite
- Minor swelling and erythema at venom injection site with formation of blister
- Ulceration of skin at injection site within 7–14 days
- Systemic symptoms of fever/chills, nausea/vomiting, and seizure are rare but do occur
- Ulcerated wound may need excision and debridement and eventual skin grafting. Healing is slow. Administration of antibiotics and corticosteroids may be helpful.

Snake Bites

Etiology
- Envenomation from pit viper or elapid snake

Nursing Diagnoses
- Pain
- Impaired skin integrity
- Risk for infection

Common Complaints
- Known snake bite, pain, nausea

Triage Rating
- Urgent to emergent

Related Factors
- The majority of poisonous snake bites in the United States are from the pit vipers. The venom contains proteolytic enzymes, toxic proteins, and cytolytic enzymes. Complications include allergic reactions, compartmental syndrome if bite occurs on the extremities, and bleeding abnormalities.

Assessment Findings
- Presence of fang marks
- Edema at site of envenomation and subsequent progression of edema
- Ecchymosis at site of envenomation
- Possible pulmonary edema
- Possible seizure activity

Diagnostics
- PT and PTT studies: may be elevated

Interventions
- Immobilize affected extremity.
- Remove constricting jewelry distal to envenomation site.
- Measure circumference of bitten extremity at site.
- Insert IV and infuse NS fluid.
- Obtain blood samples for PT, PTT, and other studies.
- If progressive swelling, administer antivenin IV infusion.*
- Administer **dT** 0.5 mL IM as needed.
- Monitor progressive swelling, BP, pulse rate and rhythm, respiratory rate, pulse oximetry, antivenin reactions.

*Antivenin Administration
- Perform a skin or eye conjunctival test of antivenin.
- Administer antivenin via slow IV infusion according to degree of swelling:

Local swelling, no systemic symptoms	3–5 vials
Progressive swelling, mild systemic symptoms	8–10 vials
Severe swelling, severe systemic symptoms	15–20 vials

Disposition   Hospital admission is required if antivenin has been administered.

Marine Life Hazards

Stingray and Scorpion Fish

- Intense local pain and swelling following sting; pain radiates centrally
- Systemic symptoms may appear in approximately 30 minutes:
  - Nausea/vomiting
  - Weakness
  - Diaphoresis
  - Vertigo
  - Tachycardia
  - Muscle cramps
- Treatment: immerse wound in hot water (115–125°F). Administer **dT** as needed and oral antibiotic **trimethoprim-sulfamethoxazole**.

Portuguese Man-of-War

- Sting, instant burning, red rash on areas where tentacles came in contact with skin
- Systemic symptoms may appear in 4–8 hours:
  - Headache
  - Lethargy, vertigo, ataxia, seizures, coma
  - Vomiting
  - Dysphagia
  - Cardiac dysrhythmia, bronchospasm, respiratory failure
- Treatment: rinse wound areas with seawater or saline, do not rub. Irrigate wound with vinegar or rubbing alcohol. Remove remaining nematocysts by applying shaving cream and shave area with razor blade. Consider administration of **dT** if open wound areas, and **prednisone** 60 mg PO for allergic reaction. Systematic symptoms are managed with supportive treatment.

Scrombroid Poisoning

- Occurs with ingestion of toxic fish: commonly albacore, tuna, mackerel, bonito, kingfish, wahoo, dolphin, sardine, anchovy, amberjack, and ocean salmon
- Symptoms occur within 15–90 minutes following ingestion:
  - Flushing of face, neck, and torso
  - Urticaria, pruritus, angioedema
  - Abdominal cramps, diarrhea, nausea/vomiting
- Treatment: for mild reaction administer **diphenhydramine** 25–100 mg PO or IM. For severe reaction administer **epinephrine** 0.3–0.5 mg 1:1000 solution SC.

Diabetic Ketoacidosis

Etiology
- Insulin production deficit

Nursing Diagnoses
- Fluid volume deficit
- Altered tissue perfusion

Common Complaints
- Nausea/vomiting, increased urination, fever, increased thirst, weight loss

Triage Rating
- Urgent to emergent

Related Factors
- A complication that occurs in individuals with inadequately treated insulin-dependent diabetes. Ketoacidosis can occur from undiagnosed diabetes or acute stress in the known diabetic individual. Sudden increases in growth or exercise can produce this stress, as can infection, or noncompliance with medication regimens. Whatever the cause, the insulin deficit produces hyperglycemia, lipolysis, and protein catabolism. The entry of glucose into the cellular structures is blocked, leading to an increase in serum glucose, osmotic diuresis, and systemic dehydration.

Assessment Findings
- Restlessness or decreased level of consciousness
- Tachycardia
- Hypotension
- Tachypnea and hyperventilation
- Possible smell of acetone on breath
- Dry, warm skin

Diagnostics
- Serum chemistries: glucose >300 mg/dl; potassium may be normal or decreased, decreased sodium
- CBC: elevated WBC because of stress or infection possible
- ABG: pH <7.35 (acidosis); $Paco_2$ <35 mm Hg (respiratory alkalosis); HCO_3 <22 mm Hg (metabolic acidosis)
- Urinalysis: increased glucose, positive ketones
- Serum acetone: elevated
- Serum osmolarity: increased

Interventions
- Administer oxygen 6–15 L via face mask.
- Insert IV and infuse NS fluid.*
- Obtain blood samples for CBC, chemistries, ABG, and other laboratory studies.
- Insert nasogastric tube and attach to suction.
- Consider insertion of indwelling urinary catheter.
- Administer medications:
  –**Regular insulin** 0.1 U/kg IV infusion.
  –**Potassium** 10–20 mEq/L IV infusion.
  –Consider **sodium bicarbonate** 50 mL IV infusion if pH <6.9.
- Monitor level of consciousness, BP, pulse rate and rhythm, respiratory rate, pulse oximetry, serum glucose, urinary output, nasogastric tube output.

*Fluid resuscitation recommendations:

1L/h of NS until BP is stabilized and urinary output is a minimum of 60 mL/h. This may necessitate 3–5 L of NS solution within the first several hours. In children the rate of infusion is 20 mL/kg bolus, then maintenance of 20 mL/kg/h. Once the serum glucose is approximately 250 mg/dl, 5% dextrose should be added to the IV solution.

Disposition   Admission to critical care or medical area.

Hyperosmolar, Hyperglycemic, Nonketotic Coma

Etiology
- Insulin production deficit

Nursing Diagnoses
- Fluid volume deficit
- Altered tissue perfusion

Common Complaints
- Vomiting, increased urination, confusion, increased thirst, fever

Triage Rating
- Emergent

Related Factors
- This condition is a complication of noninsulin-dependent diabetes. It is more common in the elderly population and carries a high mortality rate. It almost always is associated with a severe illness as the precipitating factor. As serum glucose levels increase, ketone production does not occur. Reasons for this still remain unclear.

Assessment Findings
- Restlessness, confusion, coma
- Increased temperature
- Tachycardia
- Hypotension
- Tachypnea
- Dry skin with poor turgor

Diagnostics
- Serum chemistries: glucose >800 mg/dl, decreased potassium, decreased sodium
- ABG: pH 7.35–7.34
- Serum ketones: normal
- CBC: elevated WBC from stress or infection possible
- Serum osmolarity: >350 mOsm/kg
- Urinalysis: elevated glucose

Interventions
- Administer oxygen 6–15 L via face mask.
- Insert IV and infuse NS fluid.*
- Obtain blood samples for CBC, chemistries, and other laboratory studies.
- Insert nasogastric tube and attach to suction.
- Insert indwelling urinary catheter.
- Administer medications:
  - **Regular insulin** 5–10 U/h IV infusion.
  - **Potassium** 10 mEq/L IV infusion.
- Monitor level of consciousness, BP, pulse rate and rhythm, respiratory rate, pulse oximetry, urinary output, nasogastric tube output, serum glucose level.

*Fluid resuscitation recommendations:
- Initial fluid for rehydration is NS.
- Once the patient is stabilized, fluid should be changed to 0.45 NS.
- Approximately $\frac{1}{2}$ of the volume deficit should be replaced in the first 12 hours and the second $\frac{1}{2}$ in the following 12 hours.

Disposition   Admission to critical care area.

Hypoglycemia

Etiology
- Insulin production deficit, fasting, alcohol intoxication, ingestion of beta blocker medication

Nursing Diagnoses
- Altered tissue perfusion: cerebral

Common Complaints
- Restlessness, confusion, headache, blurred vision, sweating

Triage Rating
- Emergent

Related Factors
- Insulin-dependent diabetic individuals are at greatest risk for developing hypoglycemia. It is a common problem and is defined as a serum glucose level <50 mg/dl.

Assessment Findings
- Restlessness, agitation, confusion, possible seizure activity
- Possible slurred speech
- Tachycardia
- Pale, diaphoretic skin

Diagnostics
- Serum glucose: <50 mg/dl

Interventions
- Insert IV or saline lock.
- Administer medication:
  –**Dextrose 50%** 50–100 mL IV *or* **glucagon** 1 mg IM if unable to obtain IV access.
- Monitor level of consciousness, BP, pulse rate and rhythm, respiratory rate, pulse oximetry, serum glucose level.

Disposition   The majority of patients can be released to home. If the hypoglycemia is the result of acute alcohol or beta blocker medication ingestion, hospital admission may be required.

Myxedema Coma

Etiology
- Inadequate production of tri-iodothyronine (T_3), thyroxine (T_4)

Nursing Diagnoses
- Ineffective breathing pattern
- Ineffective thermoregulation
- Risk for infection
- Altered tissue perfusion

Common Complaints
- Lethargy, irregular menses in females, feeling of cold

Triage Rating
- Urgent to emergent

Related Factors
- Without adequate thyroid hormone production, the metabolic rate slows and every body organ is affected. Myxedema coma is a complication of hypothyroidism and may be precipitated by infection, hypoxia, medications, and congestive heart failure.

Assessment Findings
- Altered level of consciousness, coma
- Subnormal temperature
- Bradycardia
- Hypotension
- Facial puffiness
- Ascites
- Nonpitting edema
- Decreased deep tendon reflex response

Diagnostics
- ECG: may demonstrate low voltage QRS complex and bradycardia
- Serum T_3, T_4: decreased levels
- Serum chemistries: decreased sodium, decreased glucose

Interventions
- Administer oxygen 6–15 L via face mask.
- Support respiratory effort: may require intubation and mechanical ventilation.
- Insert IV or saline lock.
- Obtain blood samples for CBC, chemistries, T_3, and T_4 levels, and other laboratory studies.
- Assist with rewarming by warm fluid administration, warm blankets.
- Insert nasogastric tube and attach to suction.
- Insert indwelling urinary catheter.
- Administer medication to increase metabolic rate:
  - **Levothyroxine** 300–500 µg IV.
  - **Dextrose** 50 mL IV if hypoglycemia present.
  - **Hydrocortisone** 200–400 mg IV.
- Monitor level of consciousness, BP, pulse rate and rhythm, respiratory rate, pulse oximetry, temperature, urinary output.

Disposition Admission to critical care or medical area.

Thyroid Storm

Etiology
- Overproduction of thyroxine (T_4), and triiodothyronine (T_3)

Nursing Diagnoses
- Risk for decreased cardiac output
- Ineffective thermoregulation
- Risk for injury

Common Complaints
- Nausea/vomiting, shaking or tremors, diarrhea, weight loss, weakness, shortness of breath, fever

Triage Rating
- Urgent to emergent

Related Factors
- Overproduction of T_4 and T_3 results in exaggerated metabolic activity. Causes for this overproduction include Graves' disease, recent surgery, trauma, infection, or noncompliance with medicine regimen.

Assessment Findings
- Agitation, confusion, possible seizure activity
- Increased temperature
- Tachycardia
- Hypertension
- Brisk deep tendon reflex response
- Possible exophthalmos
- Possible palpable enlarged thyroid gland

Diagnostics
- ECG: will demonstrate tachydysrhythmias such as atrial fibrillation, premature ventricular contractions, or paroxysmal atrial tachycardia
- CBC: elevated WBC because of infection or stress possible
- Serum T_3 and T_4: elevated levels

Interventions
- Administer oxygen 2–6 L via nasal cannula.
- Insert IV and infuse NS fluid.
- Obtain blood samples for CBC, chemistries, T_3 and T_4 levels, and other studies.
- Insert nasogastric tube and attach to suction.
- Cool patient with hypothermic blanket/device.
- Administer medication to slow metabolic rate:
  - **Propranolol** 5 mg IV.
  - **Propylthiouracil** (PTU) 800–1200 mg PO.
  - **Potassium iodide** 3–5 drops PO 1 hour after PTU.
  - **Acetaminophen** 650 mg PO.
- Monitor level of consciousness, BP, pulse rate and rhythm, respiratory rate, pulse oximetry, temperature, urinary output.

Disposition   Admission to critical care or medical area.

Hemophilia

Etiology
- Genetic disorder

Nursing Diagnoses
- Risk for fluid volume deficit
- Pain

Common Complaints
- Joint pain or swelling, active and excessive internal/external bleeding

Triage Rating
- Urgent

Related Factors
- Hemophilia is a disease caused by a recessive gene transmitted almost exclusively by females but occurring in males. The most common type of hemophilia results from a deficiency of factor VIII. Bleeding episodes may occur following injury or may be spontaneous. Patients usually are familiar with their disease and subsequent treatment modalities.

Assessment Findings
- Possible hemarthroses especially of knee, ankle, elbow
- Possible nasal or gastric bleeding
- Possible tachycardia
- Possible hypotension

Diagnostics
- PTT study: prolonged
- PT study: normal
- Platelets: normal or elevated

Interventions
- Insert IV and infuse NS fluid.
- Obtain blood samples for bleeding studies and other studies.
- Apply ice to any extremity injury.
- Immobilize any injured extremity.
- Administer medication:
  -**Factor VIII** (dose variable):
  - Minor bleeding 10–15 U/kg IV.
  - Major bleeding 30 U/kg IV.
- Monitor BP, pulse rate and rhythm, respiratory rate, pulse oximetry, pain relief, bleeding control, and transfusion reactions.

Disposition   Patients with minor episodes of bleeding that are well controlled with ED treatment can be released to home. Other patients should be admitted to the hospital for continual monitoring and treatment.

Sickle-Cell Crisis

Etiology
- Genetic disorder

Nursing Diagnoses
- Pain
- Altered tissue perfusion

Common Complaints
- Fever; tachycardia; joint, abdominal, back pain

Triage Rating
- Urgent

Related Factors
- The disease of sickle cell is caused by genetically defective hemoglobin. This abnormal hemoglobin causes RBCs to become altered in shape and stiff when the condition of deoxygenation occurs. Vascular occlusion occurs leading to the "crisis" state. Events that may trigger this crisis include infections, hypoxemia, anxiety, and sudden changes in altitude.

Assessment Findings
- Possible increased temperature
- Tachycardia
- Hepatomegaly and possible splenomegaly (especially in children)
- Possible priapism in males
- Retinal hemorrhage
- Pulmonary crackles
- Jaundice skin color

Diagnostics
- CBC: decreased hemoglobin and elevated WBC because of infection or stress
- Reticulocyte count: increased
- Platelet count: increased

Interventions
- Administer oxygen 6–15 L via face mask if documented hypoxemia is present.
- Insert IV and infuse NS fluid.
- Obtain blood samples for CBC and other studies.
- Administer pain relief medication:
  –**Morphine sulfate** 0.1–0.15 mg/kg IV.
- Monitor BP, pulse rate and rhythm, respiratory rate, pulse oximetry, pain relief.

Disposition   If pain relief or control is achieved within 4–6 hours of ED treatment, the patient can be released to home. If pain cannot be controlled, hospital admission to a medical area should be considered for continued pain relief therapy.

Frostbite

Etiology
- Prolonged exposure to cold environment

Nursing Diagnoses
- Pain
- Altered tissue perfusion

Common Complaints
- Pain in affected extremity, decreased or loss of sensation in affected extremity

Triage Rating
- Urgent to emergent

Related Factors
- Frostbite most commonly occurs to the feet, hands, nose, ears, or cheeks. The injury may be superficial or involve deep layers of tissue. Peripheral blood flow to the affected extremity is reduced, and interstitial ice crystals begin to form. Therapy is directed toward rewarming the frostbitten tissue. Once rewarming begins, it must be continued to prevent refreezing and further tissue damage.

Assessment Findings
- Possible overall decreased body temperature
- Frostbitten area:
  –Swollen and erythemic *or* pale, white color
  –Possible blister or bleb formation containing either clear or purple bloody fluid

Diagnostics
- None

Interventions
- Administer oxygen 6–15 L with warmed humidified air via face mask.
- Insert IV and infuse warm NS fluid.
- Obtain blood samples for possible laboratory studies.
- Slowly rewarm body if overall temperature is low.
- Rapidly rewarm frostbitten area:
  –Immerse affected extremity in heated water (105–115°F) or heated whirlpool bath.
- Administer pain relief medication:
  –**Morphine sulfate** 2–10 mg IV.
- Assist with debridement of broken blisters and those containing clear fluid; leave blood-filled blisters intact.
- Apply sterile dressings to affected areas, placing padding between frostbitten toes and fingers.
- Monitor BP, pulse rate and rhythm, respiratory rate, pulse oximetry, core body temperature, pain relief.

Disposition   Admit to critical care or medical-surgical area or consider transfer to regional burn center for further treatment.

Hyperthermia

Etiology
- Prolonged exposure to hot environment, vigorous exercise

Nursing Diagnoses
- Hyperthermia
- Fluid volume deficit

Common Complaints
- Minor: sweating, swelling of hands and feet, muscle cramping, dizziness
- Major: decreased level of consciousness, coma

Triage Rating
- Nonurgent to emergent

Related Factors
- Body temperature can increase because of various factors. Fever caused by illness is a normal physiologic hyperthermic response. Heat stress from exercise or the environment can lead to the minor heat-related conditions of heat edema, heat cramps, or heat syncope. More major conditions are heat exhaustion and heat stroke. The goal is to identify the cause of the hyperthermic response and to cool the individual's body temperature.

Assessment Findings
- Minor:
  - Dependent pitting edema
  - Moist, warm skin
  - Normal to slightly elevated temperature
- Major:
  - Decreased level of consciousness, coma
  - Hypotension
  - Tachycardia
  - Increased body temperature
  - Hot skin

Diagnostics
- CBC: possible elevated WBC because of infection or stress
- Serum chemistries: possible decreased or elevated sodium and potassium levels
- Enzyme studies: possible elevated liver and CK enzymes
- Urinalysis: presence of myoglobin indicating rhabdomyolysis

Interventions
- Administer oxygen 6–15 L via face mask.
- Insert IV and infuse cool NS fluids.
- Obtain blood samples for CBC, chemistries, PT, PTT, and other studies.
- Begin cooling measures and continue until temperature 101°F:
  - Remove clothing.
  - Spray tepid mist over patient.
  - Place ice packs in external vascular areas.
  - Place patient on ice-soaked sheets or cooling blanket.
- Administer medications to prevent shivering:
  - **Diazepam** 5–10 mg IV *or* **lorazepam** 0.5–2 mg IV *or* **chlorpromazine** 10–50 mg IM.
- Insert nasogastric tube and attach to suction.
- Insert indwelling urinary catheter.
- Monitor level of consciousness, BP, pulse rate and rhythm, respiratory rate, pulse oximetry, core temperature, urinary output.

Disposition   Release to home ONLY if minor symptoms of hyperthermia were present. All other patients require hospital admission for continued monitoring and treatment.

Hypothermia

Etiology
- Prolonged exposure to cold environment

Nursing Diagnoses
- Hypothermia
- Decreased cardiac output

Common Complaints
- Confusion, "feeling cold," shivering

Triage Rating
- Urgent to emergent

Related Factors
- A core body temperature of <95°F constitutes the diagnosis of hypothermia. The spectrum of hypothermia ranges from mild to severe. Most often hypothermia occurs from accidental exposure to a cold environment without adequate protective clothing.

Assessment Findings
- Mild:
  - Confusion
  - Bradycardia
  - Temperature 93–95°F
- Moderate:
  - Coma
  - Hypoventilation
  - Bradycardia, possible atrial fibrillation
  - Hypotension
  - Cold skin
  - Temperature 86–93°F
- Severe:
  - Coma
  - Fixed/dilated pupils
  - Bradycardia or possible ventricular fibrillation or asystole
  - Apnea
  - Hypotension
  - Temperature <86°F

Diagnostics
- ECG: bradycardia; atrial fibrillation; or in severe cases presence of Osborne wave, ventricular fibrillation, or asystole

Interventions
- If asystole or ventricular fibrillation present, begin CPR and treat rhythm with defibrillation and ACLS medications.
- Remove any wet clothing from patient.
- Cover patient with warm blankets or warm with radiant heat lamps.
- Administer warmed oxygen 6–15 L via face mask.
- Insert IV and infuse warm NS fluids.
- Obtain blood samples for laboratory studies.
- Assist with aggressive rewarming techniques to raise core temperature 1–4°F/h (0.5–2°C/h):
  - Perform warm fluid lavage.
  - Perform continuous arteriovenous rewarming (CAVR), hemodialysis, or cardiopulmonary bypass.
- Insert nasogastric tube and attach to suction.
- Insert indwelling urinary catheter.
- Monitor level of consciousness, BP, pulse rate and rhythm, respiratory rate, pulse oximetry, core body temperature, urinary output.

Disposition   Release to home ONLY those patients with mild symptoms of hypothermia once rewarming has been completed. All other patients require hospital admission for continued rewarming and monitoring.

Chemical Burns

Liquid Chemicals

- Acid substances: usually produce partial-thickness burns
- Alkaline substances: frequently produce full-thickness burns
- Treatment for either substance:
  - Remove contaminated clothing.
  - Irrigate skin/eyes/hair with copious amounts of water for minimum of 30 minutes.

Powdered Substances

- Brush off skin prior to irrigation with water.

Hydrofluoric Acid

- Cover burned areas with a dressing saturated with iced 10% calcium gluconate solution or 25% magnesium sulfate *or*
- Inject 10% calcium gluconate directly into burned tissue at dose of 0.5 mL/cm^2 or 10% magnesium solution.

Phenol

- Apply polyethylene glycol to burned tissue, then irrigate with water.

Phosphorus

- Immerse burned tissue in cool water then debride tissue to remove embedded deposits. Using a 3% copper sulfate and 1% hydroxycellulose solution to deactivate the phosphorus and assist in removal has been suggested.

Decompression Sickness

Etiology
- Rapid ascension from deep water diving

Nursing Diagnoses
- Impaired gas exchange
- Altered tissue perfusion

Common Complaints
- Chest or joint pain, rash, shortness of breath

Triage Rating
- Urgent

Related Factors
- Deep water divers using self-contained underwater breathing apparatus (SCUBA) are at risk for developing nitrogen illness and air emboli if they ascend too rapidly. Individuals may require treatment in a decompression chamber. Clinical advice on treating diving conditions can be obtained from the National Diving Accident Network (DAN), Duke University, North Carolina (919) 684–8111 or (919) 684–2948.

Assessment Findings
- Air embolus:
  - Restlessness, possible seizure
  - Diminished lung sounds because of pneumothorax
  - Pulse oximetry <94%
- Nitrogen illness:
  - Cough
  - Pulse oximetry <94%
  - Skin rash or mottling

Diagnostics
- Radiographic studies: chest film may demonstrate a pneumothorax

Interventions
- Administer oxygen 6–15 L via face mask.
- Place patient in left lateral Trendelenburg's position.
- Insert IV and infuse NS fluids.
- Monitor level of consciousness, BP, pulse rate and rhythm, respiratory rate, pulse oximetry, urinary output.

Disposition   Transfer to decompression chamber for further treatment.

High-Altitude Illness

Etiology
- Exposure to increased altitude

Nursing Diagnoses
- Impaired gas exchange
- Altered tissue perfusion: cerebral

Common Complaints
- HAPE: dry cough, shortness of breath, chest pain within 6–36 hours
- HACE: headache, confusion, ataxia, weakness, shortness of breath

Triage Rating
- Urgent

Related Factors
- Exposure to altitudes >8000 feet in unacclimated individuals can result in two high-altitude illnesses: High-altitude pulmonary edema (HAPE) and high-altitude cerebral edema (HACE). Risk factors include obesity, exertion at high altitude, and rapid altitude assent.

Assessment Findings
- HAPE:
  - Pulse oximetry <94%
  - Pulmonary wheezes or rales
  - Skin cyanosis
  - Tachycardia
- HACE:
  - Confusion and possible seizure activity
  - Tachycardia

Diagnostics
- ECG: tachycardia

Interventions
- Administer oxygen 15 L via face mask.
- Immediate descent to lower altitude.
- Administer medications:
  - **Dexamethasone** 4–6 mg PO for HACE.

Disposition   Consider hospital admission, especially if symptoms do not abate with oxygen administration and altitude descent.

Unit XIII

Toxicologic-Psychological Conditions

Alcohol Intoxication

Etiology
- Prolonged or rapid alcohol ingestion

Nursing Diagnoses
- Risk for poisoning
- Altered nutrition

Common Complaints
- Confusion, inability to walk, vomiting, shaking

Triage Rating
- Urgent to emergent

Related Factors
- Alcohol ingestion is the most common type of intoxication encountered in the ED setting. There is no one level of serum alcohol that denotes intoxication because of individual variations and chronicity of use. Patients who are long-term abusers of alcohol are at risk for sustaining chronic subdural hematomas.

Assessment Findings
- Confusion, decreased level of consciousness, coma
- Ataxia
- Tachycardia
- Slurred speech
- Alcohol odor

Diagnostics
- Alcohol level: elevated
- ABG: pH <7.35 (acidosis), Pco_2 35–45 mm Hg (normal), HCO_3 <22 mm Hg (metabolic acidosis)
- Serum glucose: may be decreased
- Radiographic studies: because of the possibility of a subdural hematoma, brain CT scan if level of consciousness does not improve over a 4-hour period

Interventions
- Assist with maneuvers to maintain a patent airway.
- Consider administering oxygen at 2–6 L via nasal cannula.
- Insert IV and infuse NS fluid.
- Administer nutritional medications:
  - **Dextrose** 50 mL IV only if serum glucose levels <50 mg/dl.
  - **Thiamine** 100 mg in 1000 mL NS.
  - **Magnesium sulfate** 2 g in 1000 mL NS.
  - **Multivitamins** 1 ampule in 1000 mL NS.
- Monitor level of consciousness, BP, pulse rate and rhythm, respiratory rate, pulse oximetry, urinary output, serial alcohol level.

Disposition   Release to home if level of consciousness improves as alcohol is metabolized. If no improvement in level of consciousness, hospital admission to critical care or medical area is required. Individuals released to home should be given information regarding detoxification and outside counseling centers.

Alcohol Withdrawal

Etiology
- Sudden decrease in alcohol consumption

Nursing Diagnoses
- Altered nutrition
- Risk for injury

Common Complaints
- Headache, nausea/vomiting, shaking, hallucinations

Triage Rating
- Urgent

Related Factors
- The symptoms associated with alcohol withdrawal occur when the individual either suddenly stops or experiences a relative decrease in alcohol intake. Symptoms may also follow a binge of alcohol intake. Mild symptoms usually begin in 6–12 hours and may be followed by seizure activity and hallucinations within 36 hours.

Assessment Findings
- Restlessness, agitation, possible seizure
- Tremors
- Tachycardia

Diagnostics
- Alcohol level: may be 0 or level may indicate a decreased concentration for the individual
- Serum glucose: may be decreased
- ABG: pH <7.35 (acidosis), P_{CO_2} 35–45 mm Hg (normal), HCO_3 <22 mm Hg (metabolic acidosis)

Interventions
- Insert IV and infuse NS fluid.
- Restrain patient as necessary.
- Administer anticonvulsant medication:
  –**Chlordiazepoxide** 25–100 mg IV/IM *or* **lorazepam** 0.5–2 mg IV/IM.
  –**Diazepam** 5–10 mg IV for seizure activity.
- Administer nutritional medication:
  –**Dextrose** 50 mL IV only if serum glucose level <50 mg/dl.
  –**Thiamine** 100 mg in 1000 mL NS.
  –**Magnesium sulfate** 2 g in 1000 mL NS.
  –**Multivitamins** 1 ampule in 1000 mL NS.
- Monitor level of consciousness, BP, pulse rate and rhythm, respiratory rate, pulse oximetry, tremor activity, urinary output.

Disposition   Admission to critical care or medical area.

Toxic Ingestions/Poisonings

- Individuals may be exposed to toxic substances through ingestion, inhalation, injection, or skin absorption. The types of substances are varied, as are the signs and symptoms patients may demonstrate.

- The overall goals in treatment are to hemodynamically stabilize the patient, identify the toxic substance, and minimize further absorption. With inhaled substances this may be accomplished via high oxygen administration; ingested substances via administration of activated charcoal and a cathartic orally or by the nasogastric route; injected substances via administration of specific antagonist medications if available; and skin absorption via removal of the toxic substance through irrigation.

- Activated charcoal dose is 0.5–1 g/kg up to 30–90 g orally. Activated charcoal with sorbitol should be avoided in children because of sorbitol's ability to overstimulate the bowel and lead to excessive diarrhea.

- Syrup of ipecac is administered only in limited cases — if the ingestion has been within 30 minutes and is a mild ingestion. The dose is 15 mL for children and 30 mL for adults. If emesis does not occur following 2 doses, gastric lavage is required.

Specific Antidote Therapies

Substance	Treatment
• Acetaminophen	• Level <150 mg/kg at 4 hours: **activated charcoal** and cathartic PO • Level >150 mg/kg at 4 hours: **N-acetylcysteine** 140 mg/kg mixed with citrus juice or soda
• Benzodiazepine	• **Flumazenil (Romazicon)** 1–3 mg IV up to 10 mg
• Beta-adrenergic blocker	• Fluids for hypotension, **glucagon** 100–150 µg/kg IV followed by 2–5 mg/h IV infusion
• Botulism	• Ingested: bivalent or trivalent antitoxin 1 ampule IM and 1 ampule IV; repeat in 4 hours • Wound: **Penicillin G** 300,000 U/kg IV infusion
• Calcium channel blockers	• **Calcium chloride** 5–10 mL (Peds: 0.1–0.2 mL/kg) IV *or* **calcium gluconate** 10–20 mL IV (Peds: 0.2–0.4 mL/kg)
• Carbon monoxide	• High-flow oxygen, possible hyperbaric chamber
• Caustic/hydrocarbon ingestions	• Oral dilution with milk or water: do not produce stomach bloating or induce emesis
• Cyanide	• Inhaled **amyl nitrate** ampules, **sodium nitrate** IV infusion, **sodium thiosulfate** IV infusion (all contained in cyanide antidote kit)
• Heparin	• **Protamine sulfate** 1 mg/100 U of heparin overdose IV
• Iron	• **Deferoxamine** 80 mg/kg IV/IM
• Isoniazid	• **Pyridoxine** (vitamin B$_6$) IV in dose equivalent to amount ingested (gram for gram); for unknown amount ingested, 5 g IV over 3–5 minutes, then repeat q3–5min until any seizure activity is controlled
• Lead/heavy metals	• **Dimercaprol** (BAL) 3–5 mg/kg IM
• Methanol/ethylene glycol	• **50% ethanol** 0.7 g/kg *or* 7 mL/kg of **10% ethanol** IV. Continuous IV infusion of 0.07 to 0.1 g/kg/h to maintain blood ethanol concentration between 100 and 200 mg/dl
• Methemoglobinemia (drug-induced)	• **Methylene blue** 1–2 mg/kg (or 0.2 mL/kg of 1% solution) IV over 5 minutes; may need to repeat dose in 1 hour
• Opiate	• **Naloxone** 2 mg IV; some opiate overdoses may require higher doses
• Organophosphate	• **Atropine** IV; large doses (up to 2 g) until secretions dry, tachycardia occurs, pupils dilate
• Phenothiazine	• **Diphenhydramine** 0.5–1 mg/kg IV or **benztropine** 1–2 mg IM
• Warfarin	• **Vitamin K** 1–2 mg IV

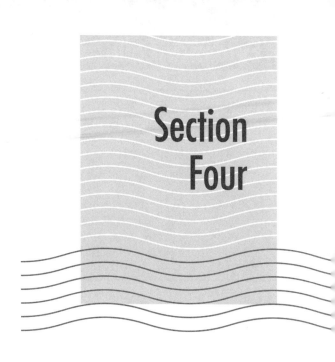

Section Four

Appendices

Evidence Collection

Evidence

- Glass fragments, bullets, broken fingernails, paint chips, loose hair follicles, fibers, or trace evidence such as soil

- Head/pubic hair

- Blood (both from venipuncture and possible hematoma evacuation), urine, gastric washings, or vomitus

- Swabs from wounds, membranes, or orifices

Collection/Container

- Place each item in a paper envelope.

- Place collection of combings and cuttings separately in a paper envelope.

- Place 20–30 mL in sealed containers.

- Air-dry prior to placing in collection container and paper envelope.

Physical Indicators Present With Child Abuse

Body Area	Injuries
• Skin	• Bruises in various distribution, age, and shape on fleshy body parts; burns with patterns of scald, immersion, iron, cigarette
• Head	• Subdural hematoma, scalp lacerations, facial/scalp hematomas, bulging fontanelle
• Eye, ear-nose-throat	• Indicators of forced feeding (bruising of gums, lips, torn frenulum), "boxing" injuries of ears, ruptured tympanic membrane without evidence of infection, retinal hemorrhages, orbital fractures, corneal abrasions
• Abdomen	• Blunt forces to midabdominal area, external signs of injury are rare
• Extremity	• Multiple fractures in various stages of healing, fractures in infants <1 year of age

Physical Indicators Present With Spousal Abuse

Body Area	Injuries
• Head, face, eye	• Intracranial hemorrhage, postconcussion syndrome, retinal detachment, altered level of consciousness, scalp and facial lacerations or bruises, facial or nasal fractures, skull fractures
• Skin	• Splash burns, friction rub burns, chemical burns, cigarette burns, knife wounds
• Abdomen	• Abdominal contusions (especially during pregnancy), miscarriage
• Musculoskeletal	• Rib fracture, back or spine injuries

Medication Infusion Rates

Dobutamine:* Infusion Rate (approximate mL/h)

Dose µg/kg/min	Body Weight in Kilograms						
	45 kg	50 kg	60 kg	70 kg	80 kg	90 kg	100 kg
1	3 mL/h	3 mL/h	4 mL/h	4 mL/h	5 mL/h	5 mL/h	6 mL/h
2.5	7	8	9	11	12	14	15
5	14	15	18	21	24	27	30
7.5	20	23	27	32	36	41	45
10	27	30	35	42	48	54	60
12.5	34	39	45	53	60	68	75
15	41	45	54	63	73	81	90
20	54	60	72	84	95	108	120

*250 mg in 250 mL D5W; usual dilution.

Dopamine:* Infusion Rate (approximate mL/h)

Dose µg/kg/min	Body Weight in Kilograms							
	45 kg	50 kg	60 kg	70 kg	80 kg	90 kg	100 kg	110 kg
2.5	5 mL/h	5 mL/h	5 mL/h	7 mL/h	7 mL/h	8 mL/h	10 mL/h	10 mL/h
5	10	10	10	15	15	16	20	20
7.5	15	15	17	23	23	25	27	30
10	17	20	25	30	30	35	40	43
12.5	20	25	30	35	37	43	45	50
15	25	30	35	40	45	53	55	60
20	35	40	45	55	60	70	80	80
25	40	50	55	70	80	90	100	100
30	50	60	70	80	90	100		
35	60	70	80	100	100			

*400 mg in 250 mL D5W; usual dilution.

Nipride:* Infusion Rate (approximate mL/h)

Dose µg/kg/min	Body Weight in Kilograms							
	45 kg	50 kg	60 kg	70 kg	80 kg	90 kg	100 kg	110 kg
0.5	7 mL/h	8 mL/h	9 mL/h	11 mL/h	12 mL/h	14 mL/h	15 mL/h	16 mL/h
1	14	15	18	21	24	27	30	33
2	27	30	36	42	48	54	60	66
3	41	45	54	63	73	81	90	99
4	54	60	72	84	96	108	120	132
5	68	75	90	105	120	135	150	165
6	81	90	108	126	144	162	180	198
7	95	105	126	147	168	189	210	231
8	108	120	144	168	192	216	240	264
9	122	135	162	189	216	243	270	297
10	135	150	180	210	240	270	300	330

*50 mg in 250 mL D5W; usual dilution.

Nitroglycerin*

Desired Dose (µg/min)	Infusion Rate (mL/h)
5	1.5
10	3
15	4.5
20	6
30	9
40	12
50	15
60	18
70	21
80	24
90	27
100	30
110	33
120	36

*50 mg in 250 mL D5W; usual dilution.

Conversion Tables

Centrigrade and Fahrenheit Conversion

C	F	C	F	C	F
0.0	32.0	35.6	96.1	37.9	100.2
26.6	80.0	35.7	96.3	**38.0**	**100.4**
27.2	81.0	35.8	96.4	38.1	100.6
27.7	82.0	35.9	96.6	38.2	100.8
28.3	83.0	**36.0**	**96.8**	38.3	100.9
28.9	84.0	36.1	96.9	38.4	101.1
29.4	85.0	36.2	97.2	38.5	101.3
30.0	86.0	36.3	97.3	38.6	101.5
30.5	87.0	36.4	97.5	38.7	101.7
31.1	88.9	36.5	97.7	38.8	101.8
31.7	89.0	36.6	97.9	38.9	102.0
32.2	90.0	36.7	98.0	**39.0**	**102.2**
32.8	91.0	36.8	98.2	39.1	102.4
33.3	92.0	36.9	98.4	39.2	102.6
34.0	93.2	**37.0**	**98.6**	39.3	102.7
34.2	93.6	37.1	98.8	39.4	102.9
34.4	93.9	**37.2**	**99.0**	39.5	103.1
34.6	94.3	**37.3**	**99.1**	39.6	103.3
34.8	94.6	37.4	99.3	39.7	103.5
35.0	**95.0**	37.5	99.5	39.8	103.6
35.2	95.4	37.6	99.6	39.9	103.8
35.4	95.7	37.7	99.8	**40.0**	**104.4**
35.5	95.9	37.8	100.0	40.6	105.0
				41.1	106.0
				41.7	107.0

Pound and Kilogram Conversion

Numbers to the far left are pounds in 10 pound increments, numbers across the top are pounds in 1 pound increments. Intersect the far left and top numbers that equal the total pounds to determine the equivalent weight in kilograms.

lb.	0	1	2	3	4	5	6	7	8	9
0	0	.45	.9	1.36	1.81	2.26	2.72	3.17	3.62	4.08
10	4.53	4.98	5.44	5.89	6.35	6.80	7.25	7.71	8.16	8.61
20	9.07	9.52	9.97	10.43	10.88	11.34	11.79	12.24	12.7	13.15
30	13.6	14.06	14.51	14.96	15.42	15.87	16.32	16.78	17.23	17.69
40	18.14	18.59	19.05	19.5	19.95	20.41	20.86	21.31	21.77	22.22
50	22.68	23.13	23.58	24.04	24.49	24.94	25.4	25.85	26.3	26.76
60	27.21	27.66	28.12	28.57	29.03	29.48	29.93	30.40	30.84	31.29
70	31.75	32.20	32.65	33.11	33.56	34.02	34.47	34.92	35.38	35.83
80	36.28	36.74	37.19	37.64	38.1	38.55	39	39.46	39.91	40.37
90	40.82	41.27	41.73	42.18	42.63	43.09	43.54	43.99	44.45	44.9
100	45.36	45.81	46.26	46.72	47.17	47.62	48.08	48.53	48.98	49.44
110	49.98	50.34	50.8	54.25	51.71	52.16	52.61	53.07	53.52	53.97
120	54.43	54.88	55.33	55.79	56.24	56.7	57.15	57.6	58.06	58.51
130	58.96	59.42	59.87	60.32	60.78	61.23	61.68	62.14	62.59	63.05
140	63.5	63.95	64.41	64.86	65.31	65.77	66.22	66.67	67.13	67.58
150	68.1	68.49	68.94	69.4	69.85	70.30	70.76	71.21	71.66	72.12
160	72.57	73.02	73.48	73.93	74.39	74.84	75.29	75.75	76.20	76.65
170	77.11	77.56	78.01	78.47	78.92	79.38	79.83	80.28	80.74	81.19
180	81.64	82.1	82.55	83	83.46	83.91	84.36	84.82	85.27	85.73
190	86.18	86.68	87.09	87.54	87.99	88.45	88.9	89.35	89.81	90.26
200	90.72	91.17	91.62	92.08	92.52	92.98	93.44	93.89	94.34	94.8
210	95.45	95.91	96.36	96.82	97.27	97.73	98.18	98.64	99.09	99.55

Pediatric Vital Signs: Normal Ranges

Age	Blood Pressure	Heart Rate (Awake) (beats per minute)	Respirations (breaths per minute)
Newborn		100–180	30–50
Infant	100-70/70-50	100–160	30–50
1–3 y	110-80/80-50	90–120	24–40
4–6 y	110-80/80-50	80–110	20–30
7–12 y	120-84/80-50	70–100	16–30
Teen	130-90/80-60	60–90	12–16

AVPU Infant Response Scale*

A—alert, responsive to environment
V—responsive to verbal stimuli
P—responsive to application of pain stimuli
U—unresponsive to stimuli

*A descriptive scale identifying the type of stimuli necessary to elicit a response in an infant.

Modified Infant Coma Scale*

Response Finding	Score
BEST EYE OPENING	
Spontaneous	4
To speech	3
To pain	2
None	1
BEST VERBAL	
Coos, babbles	5
Irritable cry	4
Cries to pain	3
Moans to pain	2
None	1
BEST MOTOR	
Normal spontaneous movements	6
Withdraws to touch	5
Withdraws to pain	4
Abnormal flexion	3
Abnormal extension	2
None	1
TOTAL SCORE	**3–15**

*Obtain best score in each category, then determine total score. Highest total score obtainable is 15, lowest is 3.

Glasgow Coma Scale*

Response Finding	Score
BEST EYE OPENING	
Spontaneous	4
To voice	3
To pain	2
None	1
BEST VERBAL	
Oriented	5
Confused	4
Inappropriate words	3
Incomprehensible words	2
None	1
BEST MOTOR	
Obeys commands	6
Localizes to pain	5
Withdraws from pain	4
Flexion to pain	3
Extension to pain	2
None	1
TOTAL SCORE	**3–15**

*Obtain best score in each category, then determine total score. Highest total score obtainable is 15, lowest is 3.

Cranial Nerves

Nerve	Function
I—Olfactory	Smell
II—Optic	Vision
III—Oculomotor	Eye movement—all eye muscles except superior oblique and external rectus. Also controls iris, sphincter, and ciliary muscles
IV—Trochlear	Superior oblique eye muscle movement
V—Trigeminal	Sensory—face, sinuses, tooth area
VI—Abducens	External rectus eye muscle movement
VII—Facial	Facial movement
VIII—Acoustic	Hearing
IX—Glossopharyngeal	Sensory—posterior area of tongue, tonsil, and pharynx. Motor—pharyngeal musculature
X—Vagus	Sensory, Motor—heart, lungs, bronchi, gastrointestinal tract, etc.
XI—Accessory	Shoulder, neck movement
XII—Hypoglossal	Tongue movement

Common Laboratory Values/Interpretations

Common Laboratory Values/Interpretations

Test	Normal Range Value	Interpretation (Possible Causes)
COMPLETE BLOOD COUNT (CBC)	VALUES MAY VARY AMONG LABORATORIES	
Hemoglobin (Hgb)	Female: 12–16 g/dl Male: 13.5–17.5 g/dl	**Increased:** dehydration, hemoconcentration, COPD **Decreased:** anemia, blood loss, overhydration
Hematocrit (HCT)	Female 37%–47% Male: 40%–54%	**Increased:** same as hemoglobin **Decreased:** same as hemoglobin
Red blood cells (RBC)	Female: 3.6–5.4 million per μL Male: 4.5–6.2 million per μL	**Increased:** polycythemia vera, dehydration, hemorrhage (during and immediately following blood loss) **Decreased:** same as hemoglobin, subacute endocarditis
White blood cells (WBC)	4100–10,900/μL	**Increased:** bacterial infection, leukemia, injury **Decreased:** aplastic anemia, immune disorders, viral infection
DIFFERENTIAL Neutrophils	45%–75% of total white blood count (WBC)	**Increased:** bacterial infections (immature cells, "bands," may be increased indicating acute infection—referred to as a "left shift"), leukemia, hemorrhage **Decreased:** viral infections, lymphoblastic leukemia
Lymphocytes	15%–45% of total WBC	**Increased:** viral infections, mononucleosis **Decreased:** bacterial infections, injury
Eosinophil	0.3%–7% of total WBC	**Increased:** allergic reactions, parasitic infestations, Addison's disease **Decreased:** congestive heart failure (CHF), Cushing's syndrome, mononucleosis
Basophil	0.3%–2% of total WBC	**Increased:** leukemia, postsplenectomy **Decreased:** acute allergic reactions, prolonged steroid therapy
Monocytes	0.6%–10% of total WBC	**Increased:** chronic infections or recovery period of acute infections, viral infections **Decreased:** prednisone therapy
ERYTHROCYTE SEDIMENTATION RATE (ESR)	Females: 0–20 mm/h Males: 0–10 mm/h	**Increased:** infection **Decreased:** CHF, sickle cell anemia
ELECTROLYTES Sodium(Na⁺)	135–145 mEq/L	**Increased:** dehydration, hemoconcentration, Cushing's disease, increased sodium intake **Decreased:** overhydration, decreased sodium intake, burns, diarrhea, vomiting, Addison's disease, diabetic ketoacidosis (DKA)
Potassium (K⁺)	3.5–5.0 mEq/L	**Increased:** renal disease, increased potassium intake, acidosis, uncontrolled diabetes **Decreased:** decreased potassium intake, use of diuretic medications, alkalosis, diarrhea, vomiting, burns
Calcium (Ca²⁺)	Total: 4.5–5.3 mEq/L Ionized: 2.1–2.6 mEq/L	**Increased:** renal disease, increased calcium intake, metastatic cancer involving bone, increased vitamin D intake, hyperparathyroidism, respiratory acidosis **Decreased:** pancreatitis, diarrhea, overhydration, hypoparathyroidism, malabsorption, alkalosis
Magnesium (Mg²⁺)	1.3–2.1 mEq/L	**Increased:** renal failure, DKA before treatment, use of antacids **Decreased:** chronic diarrhea, nutritional deficiencies, chronic alcoholism
COAGULATION STUDIES Prothrombin time (PT)	10–14 s	**Increased:** vitamin K deficiency, liver disease, anticoagulant therapy, disseminated intravascular coagulation (DIC)
Partial thromboplastin time (PTT)	30–45 s	**Increased:** hemophilia, heparin therapy, DIC **Decreased:** cancer, immediately following hemorrhage, early DIC

Common Laboratory Values/Interpretations *Continued*

Test	Normal Range Value	Interpretation (Possible Causes)
COAGULATION STUDIES	VALUES MAY VARY AMONG LABORATORIES	
Fibrin split products	–4 µL/mL	**Increased:** DIC, hypoxia, pulmonary emboli, infection, burns, some snake bites, heat stroke
Fibrinogen	Thrombin time, semiquantitative: 200–400 mg/dl	**Increased:** hepatitis, cancer, pregnancy, burns, compensated DIC **Decreased:** liver disease, DIC
Platelet count	130,000–370,000/mL	**Increased:** polycythemia vera, injury, postsplenectomy, acute infection, cirrhosis, tuberculosis **Decreased:** hemolytic anemia, following massive blood transfusions
ENZYMES	VALUES VARY AMONG LABORATORIES, DEPENDING ON TEST USED	
Alkaline phosphatase	25–92 U/L	**Increased:** liver disease, bone disease **Decreased:** malnutrition, placental insufficiency
Creatine kinase (CK) total	Females: 96–140 U/L Males: 38–174 U/L	**Increased:** damage or injury to brain, heart, skeletal muscle
Isoenzyme CK–BB	0% of total CK	**Increased:** injured cerebral tissue
Isoenzyme CK–MB	0.4–5.6 ng/mL (<2.5% of total CK)	**Increased:** myocardial injury (increases 4–6 hours post MI)
Isoenzyme CK–MM	Majority of CK	**Increased:** skeletal injury, rhabdomyolysis
Lactic dehydrogenase (LDH) total	48–115 IU/L	**Increased:** acute MI, hepatic disease, shock, cancer
LDH 1	18%–30% of total LDH	**Increased:** myocardial injury
LDH 2	30%–40% of total LDH	**Increased:** myocardial injury, MI
Serum glutamic-oxaloacetic transaminase (SGOT)	8–20 U/L	**Increased:** hepatic injury or infection (hepatitis, cirrhosis), acute pancreatitis, crush injury
Serum glutamic-pyruvic transaminase (SGPT)	Females: 9–25 U/L Males: 10–32 U/L	**Increased:** hepatic injury or infection (hepatitis, active cirrhosis)
Amylase	50–150 U/L	**Increased:** pancreatic injury or inflammation, mumps, acute cholecystitis, ruptured ectopic pregnancy **Decreased:** hepatitis, cirrhosis, toxemia of pregnancy
Lipase	2–4 U/L or 0–24 U/dl	**Increased:** pancreatitis, duct obstruction, cirrhosis, acute cholecystitis
ARTERIAL BLOOD GAS		
pH	7.35–7.45	**Increased:** hyperventilation, ingestion of alkaline substances, prolonged vomiting or gastric suctioning, compensation for acidosis **Decreased:** hypoventilation, loss of bicarbonate, prolonged diarrhea, compensation for alkalosis
$PaCO_2$	35–45 mm Hg	**Acute increase:** respiratory depression **Acute decrease:** hyperventilation
HCO_3	22–26 mm Hg	**Acute increase:** ingestion of alkaline substances, vomiting **Acute decrease:** diarrhea
PaO_2	80–100 mm Hg	**Increased:** increased supplemental oxygen **Decreased:** respiratory diseases, anemia, altitude elevation
O_2 saturation	94%–99%	**Decreased:** respiratory diseases, anemia, altitude elevation
CEREBROSPINAL FLUID	VALUES IN ADULTS (MAY VARY AMONG LABORATORIES)	
Opening pressure	50–180 mm H_2O	**Increased:** elevated intracranial pressure, meningitis
Color	Clear, colorless	**Blood:** traumatic tap (color will usually clear as fluid is collected), subarachnoid or cerebral hemorrhage (blood evenly mixed in all three tubes) **Turbid:** increased WBCs, RBCs, yeast, bacteria

Table continued on following page

Common Laboratory Values/Interpretations   *Continued*

Test	Normal Range Value	Interpretation (Possible Causes)
CEREBROSPINAL FLUID	VALUES IN ADULTS (MAY VARY AMONG LABORATORIES)	
Total cell count	0–5 WBC/μL 0 RBC	**Increased WBC:** bacterial meningitis, tuberculous meningitis, Guillain-Barré syndrome
Protein	15–45 mg/dl	**Increased:** purulent meningitis, Guillain-Barré syndrome, subarachnoid hemorrhage, aseptic meningitis
Glucose	45–85 mg/dl	**Increased:** diabetes **Decreased:** meningitis (may be normal with viral or aseptic meningitis), hypoglycemia
MISCELLANEOUS	VALUES MAY VARY AMONG LABORATORIES	
Blood urea nitrogen (BUN)	7–18 mg/dl	**Increased:** renal impairment or failure, shock, dehydration, diabetes **Decreased:** liver failure, negative nitrogen balance, overhydration
Creatinine	Females: 0.6–1.2 mg/dl Males: 0.7–1.3 mg/dl	**Increased:** renal impairment, urinary tract obstruction **Decreased:** muscular dystrophy
Uric acid	Females: 2.6–6.0 mg/dl Males: 3.5–7.2 mg/dl	**Increased:** gout, severe eclampsia, shock, alcoholism, DKA **Decreased:** allopurinol therapy
Albumin	3.8–5.0 g/dl	**Decreased:** edema, liver disease, burns, eclampsia, diarrhea, malabsorption
Plasma osmolality	275–295 mOsm/L	**Increased:** dehydration, DKA **Decreased:** hyponatremia, overhydration
Glucose (nonfasting)	85–125 mg/dl	**Increased:** diabetes, stress, pancreatitis, chronic liver disease, potassium deficiency **Decreased:** overdose of insulin, bacterial sepsis, pancreatic cancer
URINALYSIS	VALUES MAY VARY AMONG LABORATORIES	
Color	Yellow Straw color is normal: indicates low specific gravity Amber color is normal: indicates high specific gravity	**Orange:** medications (Pyridium), dehydration, bile pigment **Brownish yellow:** bile, bilirubin **Red or dark brown:** myoglobin, blood **Smoky:** blood
Specific gravity	1.003–1.035	**Increased:** dehydration, diabetes **Decreased:** diabetes insipidus, renal damage, absence of antidiuretic hormone (ADH)
pH	4.6–8	**Acid urine:** acidosis, diarrhea, dehydration **Alkaline urine:** UTI, chronic renal failure
Blood	Negative	**Positive:** UTI, subacute bacterial endocarditis, glomerulonephritis, renal calculi, crush injury
Protein	1–14 mg/dl	**Increased:** toxemia, renal calculi, renal disease, trauma, liver disease
Glucose	Negative	**Positive:** following a heavy meal, low tubular reabsorption rate, diabetes
Ketones	Negative	**Positive:** fever, diabetic ketoacidosis, prolonged vomiting, diarrhea, fasting
Nitrate/bacteria	Negative A high specific gravity of urine may yield a false negative result	**Positive:** UTI
Leukocyte esterase	Negative	**Positive:** pyuria Vaginal discharge and trichomonas may yield a false positive result
Bilirubin	<0.2 mg/dl	**Increased:** hepatitis or other liver disease, biliary tract disease
Cells and casts (microscopic)	WBC: 0–4/high-power field WBC casts: none Epithelial cells/casts: few Hyaline, granular casts: few	**Increased:** WBC—bacterial infection WBC casts—renal infection Epithelial cells/casts—nephrosis, poisoning from heavy metals Hyaline casts—fever, strain or exercise Granular casts—pyelonephritis, acute tubular necrosis, chronic lead poisoning
Crystals (microscopic)	Acid urine: urate, uric acid, calcium oxalate substances Alkaline urine: calcium phosphate, amorphous phosphate substances	**Abnormal substances:** cystine, leucine, cholesterol, sulfonamide

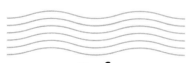

References

Birnbaum JS: The Musculoskeletal Manual. 2nd ed. Philadelphia, Saunders.

Christopher NC: Current therapeutic guidelines: Antimicrobial therapy in the pediatric patient. Emerg Med Reports 16(8): 71–77, 1995.

Englanoff G, Anglin D, Hutson HR: Lisfranc fracture-dislocation: A frequently missed diagnosis in the emergency department. Ann Emerg Med 26:229–233, 1995.

Green SM: Acute pharyngitis: The case for empiric antimicrobial therapy. Ann Emerg Med 25:404–406, 1995.

Ho MT, Saunders CE (eds): Current Emergency Diagnosis and Treatment. 3rd ed. Norwalk, CT, Appleton & Lange, 1990.

Kitt S, Selfridge-Thomas J, Proehl J, Kaiser J (eds): Emergency Nursing: A Physiologic and Clinical Perspective. 2nd ed. Philadelphia, Saunders, 1995.

Klein AR, Lee G, Manton A, et al (eds): Emergency Nursing Core Curriculum. 4th ed. Philadelphia, Saunders, 1994.

Labus JB (ed): The Physician Assistant Medical Handbook. Philadelphia, Saunders, 1995.

Mengel MB, Schwiebert LP (eds): Ambulatory Medicine: The Primary Care of Families. Norwalk, CT, Appleton & Lange, 1993.

Pichichero ME: Group A streptococcal tonsillopharyngitis: Cost-effective diagnosis and treatment. Ann Emerg Med 25:390–403.

Roberts JR: Corneal abrasions: Potential for serious morbidity. Emerg Med News 9+, 1995.

Selfridge-Thomas J: Manual of Emergency Nursing. Philadelphia, Saunders, 1995.

Tarascon Pocket Pharmacopoeia. Loma Linda, CA, Tarason, 1996.

Uphold CR, Graham MV: Clinical Guidelines in Family Practice. 2nd ed. Gainesville, FL, Barmarrae Books, 1994.

Index

Pulmonary edema, 82
  high-altitude, 185
Pulmonary embolism, 83
Pyelonephritis, 126
Pyloric stenosis, 115

R

Radial head, subluxation of, 147
Radius, fracture of, 146
Rash, fungal, 161
  hypersensitivity, 162
  infestation, 163
  viral, 160
Red blood cells, 204
Renal calculi, 127
Retina, detachment of, 55
Retinal artery, central, occlusion of, 46
Ribs, fracture of, 84
Rickettsia rickettsii, 166
Rocky Mountain spotted fever, 166
Roseola, 160
Rotator cuff tear, 141
Rubella, 160
Rubeola, 160

S

Scabies, 163
Scarlatina, 159
Scombroid poisoning, 170
Scorpion fish sting, 170
Scrotal pain, 118
Seizure, 43
Septic arthritis, 149
Septic shock, 6
Serum glutamic-oxaloacetic transaminase (SGOT), 205
Serum glutamic-pyruvic transaminase (SGPT), 205
Sexually transmitted diseases, 125
Shock, anaphylactic, 2
  cardiogenic, 3
  hypovolemic, 4
  neurogenic, 5
  septic, 6
Shoulder, dislocation of, 147
  separation of, 140
Sickle-cell crisis, 178
Simple pneumothorax, 81
Sinus bradycardia, 95
Sinus tachycardia, 94
Sinusitis, 66
Skin, abscess of, 156
  chemical burns of, 183
  electrical burn of, 33
  injury to, 154
  thermal burn of, 32
Skull, injury to, 39
Snake bite, 169
Sodium, 204
Spider bite, 168
Spinal injury, 8
Spleen, injury to, 23
Spontaneous pneumothorax, 81
Spousal abuse, 198
Sprain, 143
Stenosis, pyloric, 115
Stingray, 170
Stings, marine, 170
Stomach, injury to, 24
Stomatitis, 69
Stroke, 37
Subacromial bursitis, 141
Subarachnoid aneurysm, rupture of, 13
Subarachnoid hematoma, 13
Subconjunctival hemorrhage, 56
Subdural hematoma, 10
Subluxation, joint, 147
Subungual hematoma, 155

Suicide, 193
Sutures, 154
Syphilis, 125
Syrup of ipecac, 190

T

Tachycardia, atrial, paroxysmal, 96
  sinus, 94
  ventricular, 104
Tarsometatarsal fracture, 146
Tendinitis, upper extremity, 141
Tendon, rupture of, 144
Tenosynovitis, upper extremity, 141
Tension headache, 38
Tension pneumothorax, 19
Testes, inflammation of, 121
  torsion of, 122
Tetanus prophylaxis, 154
Thermal burn, 32
Thorax, blood in, 20
Thumb, fracture of, 146
Thyroid hormones, 175, 176
Thyroid storm, 175
Thyroxine (T_4), 175, 176
Tibia, fracture of, 146
Tietze's syndrome, 85
Tinea, 161
Toe, fracture of, 146
Toenail, ingrown, 164
Tonsillitis, 68
Toxic ingestion, 190
Trachea, injury to, 16
Tracheobronchial tree, injury to, 16
Transient ischemic attack, 37
Treponema pallidum, 125
Trichomonas vaginalis, 125
Trigeminal neuralgia, 44
Triiodothyronine (T_3), 175, 176
Tuberculosis, 86
Tympanic membrane, rupture of, 63

U

Ulcer, 113, 116
Ulna, fracture of, 146
Upper extremity, inflammation of, 141
  tendon rupture of, 144
Urethra, injury to, 29
Uric acid, 206
Urinalysis, 206
Urinary retention, 128
Urinary tract infection, lower, 129
  upper, 126
Urticaria, 162
Uveitis, 51

V

Varicella, 160
Ventricular fibrillation, 105
Ventricular tachycardia, 104
Vincent's stomatitis, 69
Viral exanthem, 160
Viral rash, 160
Vital signs, pediatric, 202

W

Warfarin, antidote for, 191
White blood cells, 204
Wound management, 154
Wrist sprain, 143
Wrist tendinitis, 141

Y

Yergason test, 144